Prescribing at a Glance

Sarah Ross

MBChB, FRCP, MD, MSc Clinical
Pharmacology, MMed
NHS Grampian/University of Aberdeen
Aberdeen, UK

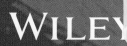

WILEY Blackwell

This edition first published 2014 © 2014 John Wiley & Sons, Ltd

Registered Office
John Wiley & Sons Ltd, The Atrium, Southern Gate, Chichester, West Sussex, PO19 8SQ, UK

Editorial Offices
350 Main Street, Malden, MA 02148-5020, USA
9600 Garsington Road, Oxford, OX4 2DQ, UK
The Atrium, Southern Gate, Chichester, West Sussex, PO19 8SQ, UK

For details of our global editorial offices, for customer services, and for information about how to apply for permission to reuse the copyright material in this book please see our website at www.wiley.com/wiley-blackwell.

The right of Sarah Ross to be identified as the author of this work has been asserted in accordance with the UK Copyright, Designs and Patents Act 1988.

Library of Congress Cataloging-in-Publication Data is available
9781118257319

A catalogue record for this book is available from the British Library.

Cover image: Science Photo Library © Mark Thomas/Science Photo Library
Cover design by Meaden Creative

Set in 9.5/11.5pt MinionPro by Toppan Best-set Premedia Limited
Printed and bound in Singapore by Markono Print Media Pte Ltd

1   2014

Contents

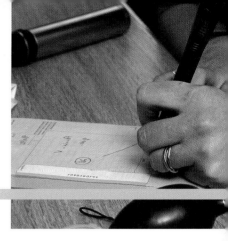

Part 5 **Specific drug groups 51**

Preface

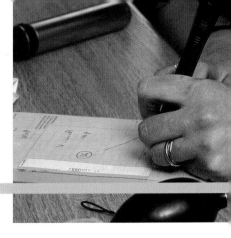

Prescribing is a core skill for all doctors, and increasingly for non-medical staff. It is a difficult skill to learn. A great deal of attention has been paid to prescribing skills in recent times, and the new Prescribing Safety Assessment has focussed minds on ensuring that new graduates are ready to prescribe safely. I hope that this book will be helpful to students and doctors learning to prescribe. As with many skills, practice is essential, and you should take every opportunity to plan the exact prescription of a drug for patients that you see. *Prescribing Scenarios at a Glance* provides useful practical examples to work through that are referenced within this text. This book has been written with new graduates embarking on the Foundation Programme in mind, and therefore focuses on mainly hospital-related prescribing; however, many of the principles extend to primary care situations. A highly practical approach has been taken, but will not describe all possible ways to look at a prescribing problem. Seek out the advice of experienced colleagues, whether doctors, nurses or pharmacists, who can provide guidance to the novice prescriber.

This book is deliberately concise, and may be supplemented by *Medical Pharmacology at a Glance* which gives a useful summary of drug mechanisms of action.

Acknowledgements

Thanks to Dr Mary Joan Macleod for critical review and suggestions.

Further reading

Joint Formulary Committee (2013). British National Formulary 66th ed. British Medical Association and Royal Pharmaceutical Society of Great Britain, London.

Richards D, Coleman J, Reynolds J, Aronson J (2011). Oxford Handbook of Practical Drug Therapy. Oxford University Press, Oxford.

Nicholson TRJ, Singer DRJ (eds) (2014). Pocket Prescriber. CRC Press, London.

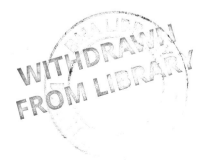

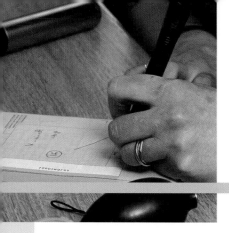

How to use your textbook

Features contained within your textbook

Each topic is presented in a double-page spread with clear, easy-to-follow diagrams supported by succinct explanatory text.

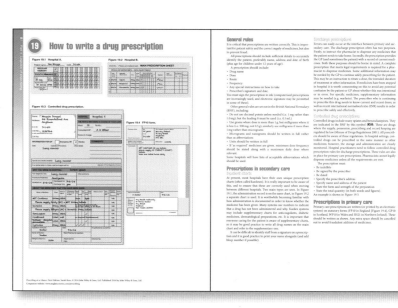

Your textbook is full of **illustrations and tables**.

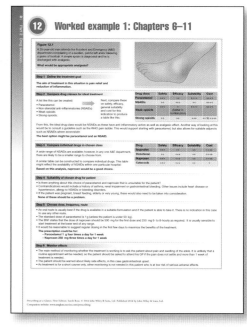

The anytime, anywhere textbook

Wiley E-Text

Your book is also available to purchase as a **Wiley E-Text: Powered by VitalSource** version – a digital, interactive version of this book which you own as soon as you download it.

Your **Wiley E-Text** allows you to:

Search: Save time by finding terms and topics instantly in your book, your notes, even your whole library (once you've downloaded more textbooks)

Note and Highlight: Colour code, highlight and make digital notes right in the text so you can find them quickly and easily

Organize: Keep books, notes and class materials organized in folders inside the application

Share: Exchange notes and highlights with friends, classmates and study groups

Upgrade: Your textbook can be transferred when you need to change or upgrade computers

Link: Link directly from the page of your interactive textbook to all of the material contained on the companion website

The **Wiley E-Text** version will also allow you to copy and paste any photograph or illustration into assignments, presentations and your own notes.

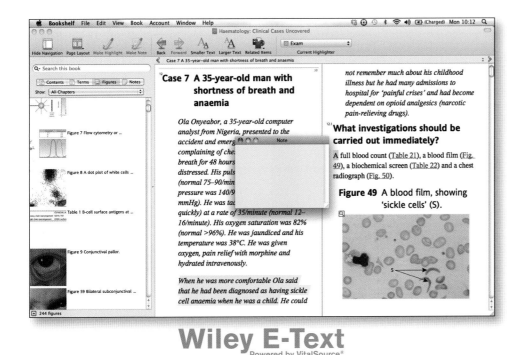

To access your Wiley E-Text:

- Visit **www.vitalsource.com/software/bookshelf/downloads** to download the Bookshelf application to your computer, laptop, tablet or mobile device.
- Open the Bookshelf application on your computer and register for an account.
- Follow the registration process.

CourseSmart

CourseSmart gives you instant access (via computer or mobile device) to this Wiley-Blackwell e-book and its extra electronic functionality, at 40% off the recommended retail print price. See all the benefits at: **www.coursesmart.com/students**

Instructors … receive your own digital desk copies!
CourseSmart also offers instructors an immediate, efficient, and environmentally-friendly way to review this book for your course.

For more information visit ***www.coursesmart.com/instructors***.

With CourseSmart, you can create lecture notes quickly with copy and paste, and share pages and notes with your students. Access your **CourseSmart** digital book from your computer or mobile device instantly for evaluation, class preparation, and as a teaching tool in the classroom.

Simply sign in at **http://instructors.coursesmart.com/ bookshelf** to download your Bookshelf and get started. To request your desk copy, hit 'Request Online Copy' on your search results or book product page.

We hope you enjoy using your new book. Good luck with your studies!

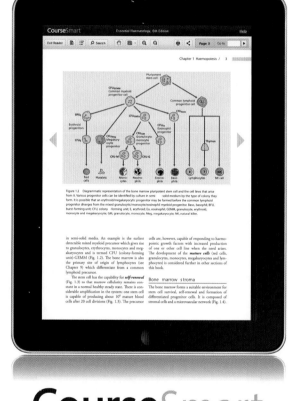

About the companion website

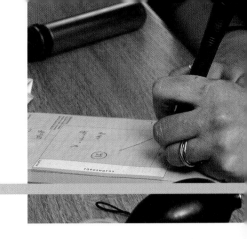

Don't forget to visit the companion website for this book:

www.ataglanceseries.com/prescribing

There you will find valuable material designed to enhance your learning, including:

- Interactive multiple-choice questions
- Case studies to test your knowledge

Scan this QR code to visit the companion website.

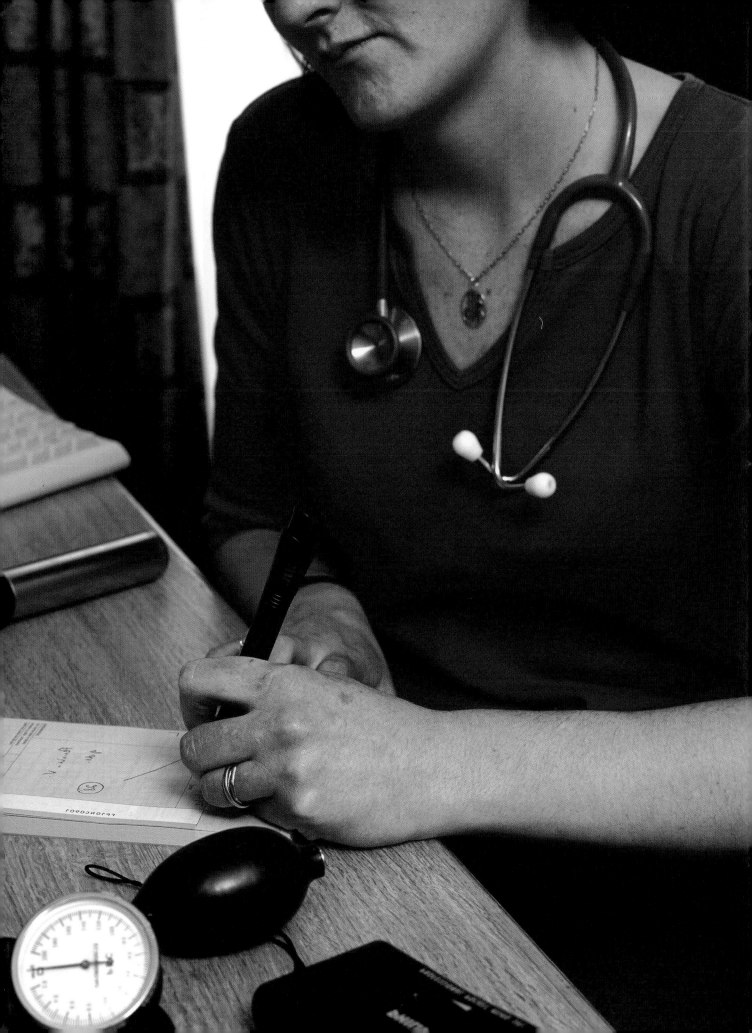

Basic principles of prescribing

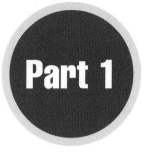

Part 1

Chapters

Don't forget to visit the companion website for this book
www.ataglanceseries.com/prescribing to do some
practice MCQs and case studies on these topics.

1 Introduction: principles of good prescribing

Box 1.1 Prescribing framework

Ideally, you should build up a 'personal formulary' of drugs for common situations.

When choosing drugs to use consider the following:
- What is the diagnosis?
- What are you trying to achieve?
- Make a list of possible drug classes that could do this
- Compare them according to safety, efficacy, suitability and cost
- Select a first-choice drug class for this situation
- Compare drugs within the class in the same way
- Select a first-choice drug for this situation

When you are treating a patient with this type of problem:
- Ensure that you have defined the patient's problem and specified the therapeutic objective
- Consider your first-line drug from your personal formulary (or go through the steps above)
- Check suitability of the first-choice drug for this patient: Is it likely to be effective? Is it likely to be safe? Is the form and dose suitable? Is the duration suitable?
- If so, start treatment. If not, reconsider. Would a change to the standard regimen for the drug help? Would a different drug from the same class be suitable? Do you need to go back to the beginning of the process and select a different drug class for this patient?
- Once a drug and regimen is selected, start treatment
- Give information to the patient
- Monitor/stop treatment as appropriate

Worked examples can be found in Chapters 12 and 13.

Prescribing at a Glance, First Edition. Sarah Ross. © 2014 John Wiley & Sons, Ltd. Published 2014 by John Wiley & Sons, Ltd.
Companion website: www.ataglanceseries.com/prescribing

Prescribing is more than writing a drug order on a chart and requires a subset of competencies involving knowledge, judgement and skill. These skills include medication history taking, reviewing medicines, choosing a new medicine, assessing the suitability of a drug regimen for a patient, writing a prescription, communicating with a patient about their medicines, monitoring drug effects, and dealing with drug-related problems. Prescribing is currently undertaken in a complex healthcare environment with growing numbers of medicines, ageing patients who have increasing numbers of comorbidities, and dwindling resources. Studies have highlighted adverse drug effects and prescribing errors as significant issues. These issues highlight the need for careful and thoughtful prescribing by all prescribers.

Prescribing well is difficult. Opportunities to practice as a student are limited, and looking back many doctors describe an insufficient emphasis on the practical aspects of prescribing in the undergraduate curriculum. This book is one attempt to help by providing clear, concise guidance on how to prescribe safely and effectively, and should be used in combination with practical examples. It could also be helpful as a guide for new graduates as they learn 'on the job'.

One of the ways to ensure good prescribing is to use a framework such as the one described in Box 1.1, which is based on the World Health Organization *Guide to Good Prescribing*. The steps are outlined in individual chapters of this book. As you develop from a novice into an expert prescriber, the steps will become automatic; however, there will still be times when it is helpful to deliberately work through each one to ensure a good choice is made.

Another element of learning to prescribe is to watch how established practitioners approach it, and to ask why they have selected a particular treatment regimen. This can give insight into the prescribing process, but be careful to consider their choice critically.

Be wary about drug information, particularly if supplied by the manufacturer for marketing purposes. Where possible, seek out unbiased data.

Further Reading

De Vries TPG, Henning RH, Hogerzeil HV, Fresle DA. (1994) Guide to Good Prescribing: A Practical Manual. World Health Organization, Geneva.

Revision: pharmacokinetics

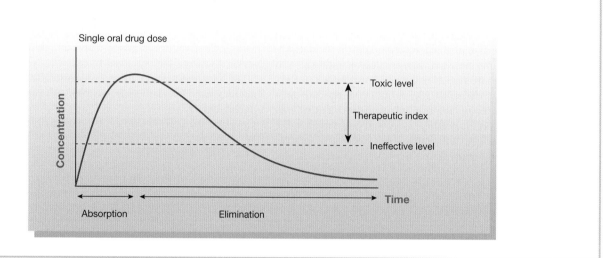

Figure 2.1 Pharmacokinetics of a single oral dose.

Prescribing at a Glance, First Edition. Sarah Ross. © 2014 John Wiley & Sons, Ltd. Published 2014 by John Wiley & Sons, Ltd.
Companion website: www.ataglanceseries.com/prescribing

Pharmacokinetics describes the way in which drugs are processed by the body through absorption, distribution, metabolism and excretion. Understanding these processes helps prescribers choose appropriate routes, doses and frequencies of admission, as well as avoid adverse drug reactions in vulnerable populations.

Absorption

In order for a drug to have its intended effect, it must reach the tissues via the systemic circulation. Bioavailability is the term used to describe the percentage of the administered drug that reaches the circulation. For the intravenous route, the bioavailability is 100%. For the oral route, bioavailability is variable as some of the drug is lost between the gut and the systemic circulation. Absorption is affected by the formulation of the drug, as well as its size, lipid solubility and ionisation. Smaller particle size, higher lipid solubility and weaker ionisation will increase absorption. Absorption is also dependent on factors in the gut (pH, motility) that can be affected by food and illness. Metabolism by gut bacteria, by enzymes in the gut or by the liver (known as first pass metabolism) can reduce the amount of drug that reaches the systemic circulation. For some drugs, such as glyceryl trinitrate (GTN), there is so much first pass metabolism that the oral route is unusable.

Other routes of administration can be affected by other factors, but the same principles apply to crossing physiological membranes (i.e. particle size, lipid solubility and ionisation).

Distribution

Once in the systemic circulation, the drug must reach the target site of action. Within the circulation, many drugs are bound to plasma proteins (primarily albumin). Only the 'free', unbound drug will be active or eliminated.

In order to maintain a drug concentration within the therapeutic index (see Figure 2.1), drug dosing must be balanced against elimination.

Various parameters can be measured for a drug, which allow dosing regimens to be planned. These are the volume of distribution, half-life and clearance. Many people find these concepts difficult and confusing. One key to understanding is to remember that these are only theoretical measurements that allow dosing regimens to be calculated. It is useful to know something about what these concepts are and how they relate to each other.

The volume of distribution is a measure of how well drugs penetrate tissues. This again relates to the drug's size, lipid solubility and ionisation. One particular physiological membrane with special properties is the blood-brain barrier, which is impermeable to many drugs.

Half-life is a measure of how long it takes for the concentration of drug within the body to fall to 50%. It is proportional to the volume of distribution, with widely distributed drugs taking longer to be eliminated from the body.

Clearance is a measure of how quickly a drug is eliminated from the body, either by metabolism or by excretion, or both. This is inversely proportional to the half-life of the drug.

Metabolism

Many drugs are metabolised, primarily to make them easier for the body to excrete. In general, this process occurs in the liver; however, metabolism also occurs in other organs, including the kidney and the lungs.

Liver metabolism takes two main forms in sequence: phase I and phase II reactions. Phase I reactions generally involve oxidation and the main enzymes are from the cytochrome P450 family. Reduction and hydrolysis reactions also occur. Phase II reactions usually involve conjugation with a compound such as glucuronide or glutathione. The aim of all these metabolic processes is to detoxify drugs and to make them more hydrophilic and ionised to facilitate excretion. Occasionally, metabolites can be toxic, or inactive 'pro-drugs' can be administered and activated by metabolism.

Metabolism can be disrupted by drug interactions and disease, and is variable with age and between different genetic groups (see Chapter 23).

Excretion

Most excretion occurs in the kidney, although a significant proportion happens through the biliary system.

Renal excretion is based on the glomerular filtration rate. Those drugs that are lipid soluble will be reabsorbed, whereas those that are hydrophilic and ionized, often as a result of metabolism, will be excreted. Some active secretion of drugs in the proximal tubule may occur. Renal damage can therefore lead to toxicity (see Chapter 15).

Certain drugs are excreted in bile but can be reabsorbed back into the enterohepatic circulation. Drugs that have been metabolised and conjugated tend not to be reabsorbed and can be excreted.

3 Using the British National Formulary

Figure 3.1 Example monograph from the *British National Formulary*.
(Source: Joint Formulary Committee 2013, p. 374. Reproduced with permission from the British Medical Association and Royal Pharmaceutical Society of Great Britain.)

374   5.1.5 Macrolides   BNF 66

hypoaesthesia, leucopenia, photosensitivity; *rarely* agitation; also reported syncope, convulsions, smell disturbances, interstitial nephritis, acute renal failure, thrombocytopenia, haemolytic anaemia, tongue discoloration

Dose

● 500 mg once daily for 3 days *or* 500 mg on first day then 250 mg once daily for 4 days; CHILD over 6 months 10 mg/kg once daily for 3 days; *or* body-weight 15–25 kg, 200 mg once daily for 3 days; body-weight 26–35 kg, 300 mg once daily for 3 days; body-weight 36–45 kg, 400 mg once daily for 3 days

● Uncomplicated gonorrhoea [unlicensed indication] (see also Table 1, section 5.1), uncomplicated genital chlamydial infections and non-gonococcal urethritis, 1 g as a single dose

● Lyme disease (see also section 5.1.1.3), typhoid [unlicensed indications], 500 mg once daily for 7–10 days (7 days in typhoid)

Azithromycin (Non-proprietary) PoM

Capsules, azithromycin (as dihydrate) 250 mg, net price 4-cap pack = £8.80, 6-cap pack = £13.87. Label: 5, 9, 23
Dental prescribing on NHS Azithromycin Capsules may be prescribed

Tablets, azithromycin (as monohydrate hemi-ethanolate) 250 mg, net price 4-tab pack = £2.85; 500 mg, 3-tab pack = £2.26. Label: 5, 9
Dental prescribing on NHS Azithromycin Tablets may be prescribed
Note Azithromycin tablets can be sold to the public for the treatment of confirmed, asymptomatic *Chlamydia trachomatis* genital infection in those over 16 years of age, and for the epidemiological treatment of their sexual partners, subject to max. single dose of 1 g, max. daily dose 1 g, and a pack size of 1 g

Oral suspension, azithromycin (as monohydrate) 200 mg/5 mL when reconstituted with water, net price 15-mL pack = £4.06, 30-mL pack = £11.04. Label: 5, 9
Dental prescribing on NHS Azithromycin Oral Suspension 200 mg/5 mL may be prescribed

Zithromax® (Pfizer) PoM

Capsules, azithromycin (as dihydrate) 250 mg, net price 4-cap pack = £7.16, 6-cap pack = £10.74. Label: 5, 9, 23

Oral suspension, cherry/banana-flavoured, azithromycin (as dihydrate) 200 mg/5 mL when reconstituted with water. Net price 15-mL pack = £4.06, 22.5-mL pack = £6.10, 30-mL pack = £11.04. Label: 5, 9

▌ CLARITHROMYCIN

Indications respiratory-tract infections, mild to moderate skin and soft-tissue infections, otitis media; Lyme disease (see also section 5.1.1.3); prevention of pertussis (Table 2, section 5.1); *Helicobacter pylori* eradication (section 1.3)

Cautions see notes above; **interactions:** Appendix 1 (macrolides)

Hepatic impairment hepatic dysfunction including jaundice reported

Renal impairment use half normal dose if eGFR less than 30 mL/minute/1.73 m²; avoid *Klaricid XL®* if eGFR less than 30 mL/minute/1.73 m²

Pregnancy manufacturer advises avoid unless potential benefit outweighs risk

Breast-feeding manufacturer advises avoid unless potential benefit outweighs risk—present in milk

Side-effects see notes above; also dyspepsia, tooth and tongue discoloration, smell and taste disturbances, stomatitis, glossitis, and headache; *less commonly* arthralgia and myalgia; *rarely* tinnitus; *very rarely* dizziness, insomnia, nightmares, anxiety, confusion, psychosis, paraesthesia, convulsions, hypoglycaemia, renal failure, interstitial nephritis, leucopenia, and thrombocytopenia

Dose

● By mouth, ADULT and CHILD over 12 years, 250 mg every 12 hours for 7 days, increased in pneumonia or severe infections to 500 mg every 12 hours for up to 14 days (see also Table 1, section 5.1); CHILD body-weight under 8 kg, 7.5 mg/kg twice daily; 8–11 kg, 62.5 mg twice daily; 12–19 kg, 125 mg twice daily; 20–29 kg, 187.5 mg twice daily; 30–40 kg, 250 mg twice daily
Lyme disease (see also section 5.1.1.3), ADULT and CHILD over 12 years, 500 mg every 12 hours for 14–21 days [unlicensed duration]; CHILD 1 month–12 years see *BNF for Children*

● By intravenous infusion into larger proximal vein, ADULT and CHILD over 12 years, 500 mg twice daily; CHILD 1 month–12 years see *BNF for Children*

Clarithromycin (Non-proprietary) PoM

Tablets, clarithromycin 250 mg, net price 14-tab pack = £3.75; 500 mg, 14-tab pack = £3.47. Label: 9
Dental prescribing on NHS Clarithromycin Tablets may be prescribed

Oral suspension, clarithromycin for reconstitution with water 125 mg/5 mL, net price 70 mL = £6.77; 250 mg/5 mL, 70 mL = £12.86. Label: 9
Dental prescribing on NHS Clarithromycin Oral Suspension may be prescribed

Intravenous infusion, powder for reconstitution, clarithromycin, net price 500-mg vial = £9.45

Klaricid® (Abbott Healthcare) PoM

Tablets, both yellow, f/c, clarithromycin 250 mg, net price 14-tab pack = £7.00; 500 mg, 14-tab pack = £11.30, 20-tab pack = £16.15. Label: 9

Paediatric suspension, clarithromycin for reconstitution with water 125 mg/5 mL, net price 70 mL = £5.26, 100 mL = £9.04; 250 mg/5 mL, 70 mL = £10.51. Label: 9

Granules, clarithromycin 250 mg/sachet, net price 14-sachet pack = £11.68. Label: 9, 13

Intravenous infusion, powder for reconstitution, clarithromycin. Net price 500-mg vial = £9.45
Electrolytes Na⁺ < 0.5 mmol/500-mg vial

◀ Modified release

Klaricid XL® (Abbott Healthcare) PoM

Tablets, m/r, yellow, clarithromycin 500 mg, net price 7-tab pack = £6.72, 14-tab pack = £13.23. Label: 9, 21, 25
Dose 500 mg once daily (doubled in severe infections) for 7–14 days

▌ ERYTHROMYCIN

Indications susceptible infections in patients with penicillin hypersensitivity; oral infections (see notes above); campylobacter enteritis, syphilis, non-gonococcal urethritis, respiratory-tract infections (including Legionella infection), skin infections (Table 1, section 5.1); chronic prostatitis; prophylaxis of diph-

Prescribing at a Glance, First Edition. Sarah Ross. © 2014 John Wiley & Sons, Ltd. Published 2014 by John Wiley & Sons, Ltd.

Companion website: www.ataglanceseries.com/prescribing

What the British National Formulary does and does not tell you

The *British National Formulary* (BNF) is a widely used reliable source of drug information produced by the British Medical Association and the Royal Pharmaceutical Society of Great Britain.

The BNF aims to provide prescribers with an up-to-date quick reference guide to prescription medicines in the UK. It does not include all medicines available for over-the-counter purchase, or alternative medicines. Guidance is produced using a combination of manufacturers' literature, regulatory information, clinical literature and published guidelines. The BNF for children is a companion volume that aims to deal specifically with paediatric drug use. Less information is included in the BNF about obstetric usage, treatments for malignant conditions and anaesthesia, which are felt to be covered by other specialist literature.

The BNF will give information about drug options, but generally not about how to choose a drug (see Chapter 6). More recently, it has included guidance from expert bodies. One example is the inclusion of the British Thoracic Society guidelines on the treatment of asthma. Prescribers may also need to refer to guidelines and local formularies.

The BNF provides guidance about dose and frequency, but may quote wide ranges from which the prescriber must choose, relying on general principles of dose selection (see Chapter 8). Specific guidance on starting doses and how to titrate a drug may be given along with suggested dose reductions for elderly patients may be supplied for some drug entries. The BNF also gives information about the drug preparations available that can help you make these decisions. Where dosage is calculated by weight, the specific calculation and/or dose by weight ranges are given.

A list of preparations by route of administration is given, but again you may need to choose between several options. The intravenous additives appendix in the BNF gives information on suitable solvents. For some drugs more detailed information about volumes and timing are given, but this is not universal. This information may be available in the literature provided with the drug, or from a pharmacist.

How to find the information you need

Newer versions of the BNF contain the major information in a single monograph. These are arranged by chapter (usually by system), with various levels of subheadings. Some drugs are discussed in more than one chapter, in which case it will be cross-referenced. Drug–drug interactions are listed in Appendix 1 of the BNF. The new version also lists the current adult advanced life support algorithm and emergency drug doses for use in non-hospital settings.

Older versions of the BNF may still be found in many workplaces. In these versions, information about specific drugs in liver disease, renal impairment, pregnancy and breast feeding are in separate appendices at the back.

The electronic BNF is arranged in a similar manner, but in an online format.

A typical monograph (Figure 3.1) will list the indications, cautions, side effects and dose (by indication), followed by information on specific preparations. The preparations section contains other useful information, such as symbols indicating that this is a prescription only medicine (POM), that this is a controlled drug (CD), this is not available for prescription on the NHS (NHS with a strikethrough), a symbol indicating that this preparation is less suitable for prescribing, and the black triangle indicating that this preparation is relatively new and so under heightened scrutiny (this indicates that adverse effects should be reported using the yellow card reporting system).

It is worth looking at the 'notes for prescribers' that often precede drug monographs. These may contain guidance from the National Institute for Health and Care Excellence (NICE) or the Committee on Safety of Medicines (SMC). Practical advice on various aspects of drug choice or use is outlined. Further advice on particular issues is given in the introductory chapters: 'guidance on prescribing' and 'emergency treatment of poisoning'. These include information on legal aspects (including prescribing controlled drugs) and on specific patient groups such as those requiring palliative care.

Other sources of information

At times it is necessary to use other sources of information. The BNF is an extremely useful guide for prescribers, but does not always include all the information required for good prescribing decisions.

Guidance on drug choice may be available in a local formulary or protocol, from national expert groups or organisations such as NICE. Clear summaries of evidence for benefit and risk may be given in this guidance or in publications such as *Clinical Evidence* from the British Medical Journal (BMJ) Group; however, this can be challenging to source and interpret for an individual patient.

Minimal information about the pharmacokinetics of a medicine is included in the BNF. If necessary, you should consult other sources such as the Schedule of Product Characteristics (SPC) produced by the manufacturer (and available at www.medicines. org.uk) or specific sources such as lists of detailed hepatic metabolism pathways. Other guidance, such as *The Renal Drug Handbook*, may give more information on using specific drugs in particular patient groups. Lists of side effects are not comprehensive and again the SPC may provide more information than the BNF. Side effects are generally listed in order of frequency and by body system, but those thought to be important may be listed first despite being rare. It can be difficult to assess the frequency of side effects from the BNF; these tend to be more clearly set out in the SPC. Drug–drug interactions may be recognised that are not listed in the BNF, and other sources of information such as *Stockley's Drug Interactions* may give different lists. However, it is likely that the BNF will cover most of the information needed in most situations.

Taking a medication history

Figure 4.1 Medicines reconciliation form.

GOODWILL HOSPITAL

Medicines Reconciliation

Patient ID label

Source of medication history: (minimum two sources)

✓ Patient	☐ Relative/carer	☐ GP phone call
☐ Patient own drugs	☐ Com pharmacist	✓ GP letter
☐ Repeat script	☐ ECS	

Other (please specify) ....

Admission medicines			Plan for medicines (doctor to complete)				Comments
Name	Dose	Freq	Continue	Amend	Withhold	Stop	
Aspirin	75mg	OD				✓	GI bleeding
Amlodipine	5mg	OD			✓		Hypotension
Simvastatin	40mg	OD	✓				
GTN spray	2 Puffs	PRN	✓				
Furosemide	40mg	OD			✓		Hypotension
Paracetamol	1g	QDS	✓				

Allergies (drug and reaction)	List any over the counter or alternative medicines
Penicillin – rash	Occasional ibuprofen
	Do medicines need further clarification? ☐ Yes ✓ No

List collected by: A Doctor	Plan approved by: A Consultant
Designation: FY1 Date: 22/2/13	Designation: Cons Date: 23/2/13

Prescribing at a Glance, First Edition. Sarah Ross. © 2014 John Wiley & Sons, Ltd. Published 2014 by John Wiley & Sons, Ltd.
Companion website: www.ataglanceseries.com/prescribing

Taking a comprehensive history

An accurate and comprehensive medication history is essential for safe and rational prescribing. Omissions and inaccuracies in the medication history may lead to medication errors in as many as two-thirds of patients admitted to hospital. Remember that medicines may be the cause of symptoms, may mask clinical signs and may alter the results of investigations.

The same skills are needed in taking a medication history as in other elements of gathering information. It is usually best to use the term 'medicines' when talking to patients rather than 'drugs', as the latter can have inappropriate connotations of illegal substances. Start with open questions, focussing down to more specific questions as needed. Closed questions may be effectively employed in clarifying particular elements of the medication history.

A good medication history should include:
- Current medicines prescribed – this should include the name, dose, frequency and route of administration along with the indication, duration of therapy and any difficulties experienced
- Medicines recently stopped and the reason why – remember that some drugs have a very long half-life and effects can still be seen some time later
- Previous adverse drug reactions – this information will be helpful in guiding future treatment
- Previous allergies with details of reaction – patients often confuse adverse reactions and allergies so it is important to establish exactly what the reaction was and whether it was a true allergy before documenting it as one
- Contraceptive pill/hormone replacement therapy use – patients often do not think to include these in a list of medicines taken so it is essential to ask specifically
- Over-the-counter medicines – again patients may not consider these important to mention so ask specifically about them
- Complementary and alternative medicines, vitamins and mineral supplements – these are widely used but patients generally do not volunteer information about them.

Patients may not remember accurate information about the names of medicines or doses. They may use generic or brand names and therefore it is helpful for prescribers to know both. Patients may be able to give other descriptions (e.g. colour and shape) and with care, descriptions can be matched using the *British National Formulary*. Pharmacists will also usually be able to identify medicines that come without packaging (e.g. unlabelled dosette boxes). At times, examination of packaging can be enlightening, for example if a patient keeps new medicines in an old container that has out of date directions.

Similarly, patients may struggle to recall the reason a drug was started, or when this occurred. Both pieces of information may be important. Indication may be decipherable from information such as 'for my heart' and duration can be helpful even in terms of days, weeks, months or years.

Asking about how and when medicines are taken can be useful in identifying misunderstandings or misuse (e.g. regular inhalers taken as required).

During the medication history is a good time to ask about compliance with medicines. It is thought that a patient's own report of their medication-taking behaviour may be unreliable; however, if addressed appropriately, useful information can be gained. Communicating a non-judgemental attitude is critical as patients may only give answers which they think are socially acceptable. It can help to phrase the question in a way that normalises compliance problems, for example 'Many patients struggle to remember to take all their medicines. Do you ever have difficulty with that?' Recall bias can also be an issue, so asking about a specific short recent time frame is recommended.

Medicines reconciliation and sources of information

Taking a medication history should now form the basis of a 'medicines reconciliation' process, which is designed to produce the most accurate medication list possible. Medicines reconciliation has been shown to reduce errors and readmission rates. It is now widely used at admission to hospital but is recommended for use at all changes of healthcare setting (e.g. discharge from hospital, referral to outpatient services).

A range of sources of information may be available, including verbal reports from the patient or carer, actual medicines brought along by the patient, printed lists from general practitioner records, repeat prescription slips, previous hospital records or discharge letters, and administration records from other care settings. Prescribers should be aware that a single source of information about a patient's current medication is likely to be insufficient and may be out of date. Medicines reconciliation triangulates different sources of information about a patient's medication to produce the best list. It is generally recommended that the person taking the medication history uses at least two sources to ensure an accurate list is made. There may be a delay in obtaining a second source of information, and the process may involve more than one healthcare professional. An initial history may be taken by a doctor, and a second source consulted by a pharmacist. If this is the case, it must be made clear in documentation that the process is not complete. The medicines reconciliation process usually involves the completion of a form where information sources can be documented (Figure 4.1). It also requires decisions made at this time about stopping or withholding medicines to be noted. This can be very helpful during the patient's stay or at discharge, particularly with current increases in shift working and reduction in continuity of care. Despite the attractions of this process, data suggests that it is not always used well by doctors. It is, however, widely recommended for ensuring patient safety and has been shown to decrease inaccuracies in medication lists.

5 Reviewing current medicines

Box 5.1   The NO TEARS tool

Need and indication – what is the medicine for?

Open questions – what does the patient think about it? (compliance)

Tests and monitoring – how well controlled is the disease? Are there other medicines which would be beneficial?

Evidence and guidelines – has evidence changed since the medicine was first prescribed? Is treatment in line with current best evidence?

Adverse events – is the patient experiencing side effects? Are there any potential interactions?

Risk reduction or prevention – are there other problems which can be opportunistically screened for?

Simplification and switches – can the overall medicines burden be reduced?

Source: Adapted from Lewis T. (2004) Using NO TEARS tool for medication review. *BMJ* **329**:434

Prescribing at a Glance, First Edition. Sarah Ross. © 2014 John Wiley & Sons, Ltd. Published 2014 by John Wiley & Sons, Ltd.

Companion website: www.ataglanceseries.com/prescribing

Medication review

Patients' medicines should be regularly reviewed. Reviews may be undertaken by a doctor, pharmacist or other qualified member of the multidisciplinary team. Medication review is currently particularly recommended in primary care for elderly patients with polypharmacy as studies show most are taking at least one unnecessary medicine that could be identified by regular review. Reviews should be not be restricted to the elderly or other high-risk groups. In hospital settings, review should be undertaken at key opportunities such as admission, discharge and rewriting drug charts, and is all the more important as diagnoses and treatments may be changing.

Various tools are available to aid medication review. One example is shown in Box 5.1.

Start by matching each drug to its indication. This clearly requires an accurate medication history (see Chapter 4), and may also require further information on the past medical history. Any mismatch should then be considered. If there is no indication for a medicine, it should normally be stopped (perhaps after discussion with a senior member of staff). Conditions or symptoms may change over time. It is very easy for medicines to be automatically continued despite successful treatment, particularly if the initial plan was not explicitly set out. For example, patients may continue to be prescribed warfarin on a repeat prescription long after a 6-month treatment period for venous thromboembolism has ended.

The next step is to consider the medicines that do have a current indication. Is this still the best option for the individual patient? Identify any side effects the patient is experiencing, any new conditions and their level of compliance. Then consider whether the benefits are outweighed by any side effects, risks or compliance issues. The risk–benefit ratio may have changed over time. The availability of new treatments or new evidence may also prompt reconsideration of a management plan.

Some medicines may be given to counteract the side effects of another medicine, but this should be kept to a minimum (e.g. laxatives are essential with opiates). When reviewing medicines, it is worth looking out for these and considering stopping them. It is also important to be sure that the side effect will actually respond to treatment, for example many patients taking calcium channel blockers experience swollen ankles, for which diuretic treatment is often ineffective.

In some situations, priorities in the patient's care may have changed. For example, after diagnosis of a life-limiting condition it may be more important to give medicines that increase quality of life rather than seek to prolong it by reducing the chance of other disease (e.g. statins).

High-risk medicines should be regularly reviewed using therapeutic drug monitoring (see Chapter 21).

Medication review is also a good opportunity to consider whether any potentially beneficial medicines are not currently prescribed. Evidence suggests that many risk factors and chronic diseases are undertreated.

Having said all this, medicines should not just be stopped. The patient should be informed and an explanation given. This is important to keep patients engaged in their own care and to encourage them to be aware of their medicines. You should think about how to stop the medicine. Many medicines may cause difficulties if stopped abruptly, whether through withdrawal side effects (e.g. antidepressants), unwanted 'rebound' effects (e.g. tachycardia and hypertension with beta blockers) or because time is needed for the body to readjust when a feedback mechanism is involved (e.g. corticosteroids). Information is available in the *British National Formulary*, either in the introduction to a drug class or in the individual monograph. Some guidance may be given about the length of time over which a dose should be reduced, but often you will need to make decisions about how exactly this is done. You may witness a range of different practices for specific drugs, most of which have little evidence to support them.

Junior prescribers may feel that they should not change or stop medicines started by other doctors. While it would be unwise for you to act outside your competence, it is important to remember that a patient's treatment needs are dynamic and may have changed since the medicine was last considered. Moreover, senior doctors are not infallible and may make mistakes that may need to be corrected. It may be appropriate to contact the original prescriber or the current specialist looking after the patient to discuss whether a change should be made. There are, however, situations and patients where medicines should not normally be stopped by a junior prescriber due to their complexity or serious potential consequences. A patient who has a transplanted organ taking immunosuppressant drugs is a good example where stopping medicines may be disastrous. If there is any uncertainty, discussion with another experienced prescriber may help.

Medicines review, like many aspects of prescribing, is best learned by supervised practice. You should seek out opportunities to discuss medications lists with more experienced doctors or pharmacists.

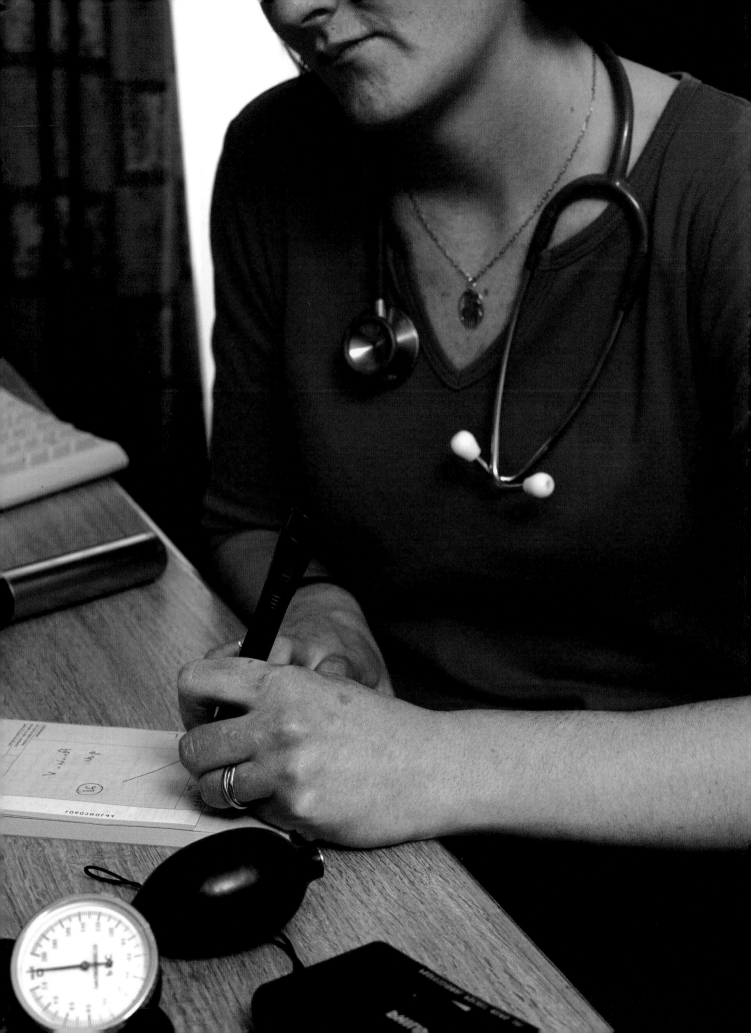

Drug selection

Chapters

Don't forget to visit the companion website for this book www.ataglanceseries.com/prescribing to do some practice MCQs and case studies on these topics.

6 How to choose a drug

What is the goal?

The first step in selecting a drug is to establish the treatment goal (i.e. what symptom or condition is being treated and what is drug therapy expected to achieve?). In some cases a diagnosis will be established, but in others the diagnosis may be less clear. In that situation it is all the more important to think about the goal of treatment. It may be to replace a substance that is missing (e.g. thyroxine), combat a disease (e.g. an antibiotic) or to alleviate symptoms (e.g. analgesia). Setting the treatment goal will help you select the most appropriate treatment and allow you to plan monitoring of treatment effects. It is always wise at this stage to consider whether drug treatment is the best way of achieving the goal.

Safety, efficacy, suitability and cost

Many prescribers learn to choose drugs based on the behaviour of their seniors or peers. While this is a convenient short-term answer, at some point it is vital that you can weigh evidence and make decisions for yourself.

The choice between options to achieve the treatment goal can be simple or complex. A system that takes into account the important factors can be useful. The World Health Organization *Guide to Good Prescribing* suggests that prescribers form their own personal formulary (a list of commonly used medicines), where they have a preferred treatment for commonly encountered situations. This idea is based on the fact that it is not practical or advisable to consider safety, efficacy and cost each time a medicine is prescribed. If this is done in advance, you will have a first-choice drug that can then be considered for an individual patient.

The first step in selecting a drug for an indication in this way is to make a list of all the possible drug classes that could be used. Drug classes should then be compared. Efficacy is often the first and most important consideration, but safety, general suitability and cost should also be considered. Usually, a balance between these factors can be struck, but at times the most effective drug will also be the safest and most cost effective. At the end of this exercise, you will have a first-choice drug class (see Chapters 12 and 13).

Next, a list of the available drugs in that class is needed. For some drug classes this is extensive, but availability may be limited by a local formulary or hospital stocking policy. Drugs in the same class may differ in efficacy, safety, suitability and cost. A similar process of comparison is needed. From this, a drug that would normally be the first choice for an indication will be selected.

You may be uncertain about where data on safety and efficacy can be found. In general, judgements should be made from published evidence in the form of clinical trials. Evidence summaries may be available in some situations. In others it may be difficult to establish the facts. You may be able to consult guidelines, whether national or local. The guideline development process is a formal way of selecting drugs by safety, efficacy and cost. Providing this is robust and unbiased, it is reasonable to trust the guideline treatment choice, perhaps even more so than using your individual judgement. Many drug trials are undertaken with select patients, and often those with multiple comorbidities or at the extremes of age are excluded. This can make judging if a treatment that has been proven in a trial will be equally efficacious and safe in an individual patient challenging. Some guidelines may have already taken this into account and may recommend different drugs for the same condition in different patient groups. Guidelines are just 'guidelines', however, and should not be followed blindly. It is perfectly justifiable to select a different treatment for an individual patient than recommended in a guideline, providing this can be explained logically. A prescriber who frequently makes choices that are not in line with guidelines may want to consider if they are really giving patients the best possible treatment.

Suitability for an individual patient

Start with your first-line agent in mind. It is imperative that you then pause to consider whether this drug is appropriate for the individual patient that you are treating. This involves considering issues such as whether there is any reason that efficacy will be different in this patient (consider, for example, age, gender and stage of illness), whether the drug is contraindicated due to a patient factor, and whether there are other considerations such as possible poor compliance.

You may need to consult the *British National Formulary* or Schedule of Product Characteristics in order to check suitability. Particular care should be taken in using a new drug in a high-risk patient such as one with hepatic or renal impairment.

In situations where the first-line drug is not suitable, you need to be clear on the reasons why in order to select an alternative drug. Some contraindications and interactions are class specific, but bear in mind that some are not. Would another agent in the same drug class be more suitable (especially in terms of convenience or type of preparation)? If not, return to the original process and decide which drug class would be the next most appropriate and which individual drug from it should be selected. Then consider its suitability in this patient.

You should take the patient's preference into account. It may be that this makes a difference to drug choice, particularly in relation to side-effect profiles or more convenient regimes.

Once the drug is chosen, further considerations about dose, frequency, route and duration can be made.

Prescribing at a Glance, First Edition. Sarah Ross. © 2014 John Wiley & Sons, Ltd. Published 2014 by John Wiley & Sons, Ltd.

Companion website: www.ataglanceseries.com/prescribing

7 How to choose frequency

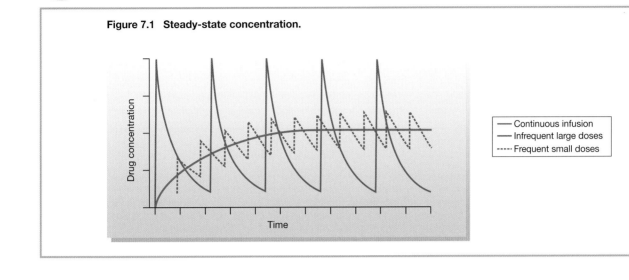

Figure 7.1 Steady-state concentration.

Continuous infusion
Infrequent large doses
Frequent small doses

Drug concentration

Time

Frequency selection

Choosing the frequency for a drug regimen is often straightforward and merely involves following the instructions given in the BNF. These tend to be set out as 'number of times per day', 'every × hours' or as a total daily dose that should be given in divided doses. A total daily dose is normally divided equally, but you should also take into account what doses are available. In general, there is a degree of flexibility in the exact timing of doses, which can be varied to suit a patient or the times of hospital ward drug rounds. It is not usually necessary to alter standard drug round times if they do not quite match the BNF, and may unnecessarily irritate nursing staff or patients. Occasionally it is important to be exact, usually where a constant concentration is desirable, for example long-acting morphine sulfate tablets (MST) for pain control (these have a 12-hour duration of action and the next dose should be given as close to 12 hours later as possible, which may not fit neatly with drug administration times in hospital).

Compliance with medicines tends to be poorer when drugs are prescribed several times a day, so where possible it is worth keeping the frequency to once or twice a day.

Changing the dose will change the steady-state plasma concentration of a drug. Changing the frequency will do the same, but remember that these are not exactly equivalent actions. Changing the dose will cause larger fluctuations in concentration than changing the frequency (Figure 7.1) and will result in more time spent outside of the therapeutic range, which may be undesirable in terms of toxicity or lack of efficacy. Some therapeutic regimens are designed around frequency rather than dose. Gentamicin once-daily dosing is a good example of this. A set dose is given (calculated by ideal body weight), and therapeutic monitoring of concentration is undertaken. If the concentration is too high, rather than reducing the dose, the frequency of administration is reduced. This should result in less toxic effects of gentamicin than varying the dose would.

Timing of dosing is also important. Mostly, patients can be encouraged to take drugs at the same time each day. Traditionally this would be in the morning, but a few drugs actually need to be given at a particular time of day. There may be instances where better control of symptoms or conditions can be achieved by varying the time of administration. For example, splitting antihypertensive therapy so that some is taken in the morning and some is taken in the evening can provide better 24-hour blood pressure control in patients who lack a normal nocturnal dip. Timing may also be important in reducing unwanted drug effects. An example of this is the prescription of diuretic drugs, where patients on twice-daily dosing may wish to take the second dose at lunchtime to avoid trips to the bathroom during the night.

Prescribing at a Glance, First Edition. Sarah Ross. © 2014 John Wiley & Sons, Ltd. Published 2014 by John Wiley & Sons, Ltd.
Companion website: www.ataglanceseries.com/prescribing

8 How to choose a dose

Box 8.1 Dose calculation examples

1. A patient needs gentamicin. The preferred dose is 7 mg/kg (i.e. the dose is calculated by body weight) and the patient weighs 59 kg.

Answer
Dose required is 7 mg × 59 = 413 mg. It is usual to round this number to the nearest multiple of 40 (gentamicin vials contain 40 mg per 1 mL), so the dose would be 400 mg (rounding down is safest practice).

However, if the patient was obese (BMI >30), their ideal body weight (IBW) should be used instead. To calculate ideal body weight (kg), use the following formula:

> For males = 50 + (0.9 for every centimetre over 150 cm);
> For females = 45.5 + (0.9 for every centimetre over 150 cm)

For example, a female patient is 160 cm (5 foot 3 inches) and 87 kg. This gives a BMI of 33.9. Ideal body weight would be 45.5 + (0.9 × 10 cm) = 54.5 kg.

So, 7 mg × 54 = 378 mg, rounded to 360 mg.

2. A patient needs an intravenous heparin infusion, to be started at 1200 units per hour. Heparin comes in 5000 units/mL (as well as a range of concentrations – do not confuse these!). The BNF states that this can be made up in 5% glucose or 0.9% saline. The infusion will need to go through a syringe pump (50 mL syringes). How do you make up the infusion and set the pump?

Answer
Make up a syringe containing 50 000 units in 50 mL. This will give you 1000 units in 1 mL (10 mL heparin using 2× 5000 units/mL 5 mL vials plus 40 mL saline)

To run at 1200 units per hour, run at 1.2 mL/hour (1 mL = 1000 units, so 0.1 mL = 100 units and therefore 1200 units will be 1.2 mL).

3. A patient presents with a stroke and needs alteplase. This should be given as 0.9 mg/kg (maximum dose 90 mg), with 10% given as an i.v. bolus and the remainder as an infusion over 1 hour. The patient weighs 83 kg.

Answer
The total dose required is 0.9 mg × 83 = 74.7 mg; 10% is 7.5 mg (rounded).
Alteplase comes with a diluent in which it should be made up. The bolus of 7.5 mg should be given. This leaves 74.7 – 7.5 = 67.2 mg to be given over 1 hour as an infusion

Prescribing at a Glance, First Edition. Sarah Ross. © 2014 John Wiley & Sons, Ltd. Published 2014 by John Wiley & Sons, Ltd.
Companion website: www.ataglanceseries.com/prescribing

Dosage selection

Once a drug is selected for an individual patient, you need to choose an appropriate dose. In some instances there is only one available dose that is suitable for all patients. This is straightforward as the dose can be found in the *British National Formulary* (BNF) or product literature. In other cases, a dose range is given in the BNF or by the manufacturer and some deliberation about dosage will be needed. This may involve the application of basic principles or a dose calculation.

In general, it is reasonable to start cautiously with the lowest available dose and increase this according to the patient's response. Many drugs that require this approach are highlighted in the BNF, where specific guidance about dose titration is also sometimes given (e.g. carbamazepine). Again this may be straightforward or more complex with instructions to check plasma concentration prior to increasing the dose. In some circumstances, you will need to consider how quickly a drug effect is needed and adapt dose titration accordingly. For some drugs, such as warfarin, there are numerous ways of approaching the situation and differing guidance can be confusing (see Chapter 28).

There are several situations where starting with the lowest dose is not appropriate. This may be because a quick response is needed or because a low dose will not be sufficiently efficacious. In these cases, you will need to choose a higher starting dose.

Selected drugs may require a 'loading' dose or doses to be given. This should be considered if a drug has a long absorption half-life, as it can take time to reach a steady-state concentration within the desired range. The loading dose(s) should produce a therapeutic concentration rapidly, after which the dose should be reduced back to a lower maintenance dose. Good examples of this approach are starting digoxin and amiodarone. Again the BNF may point this out.

Note that the same drug may be used for different indications at different doses. This can also be a source of confusion and great care is needed when checking the BNF monograph that the right indication has been selected.

Remember that the dose of a drug is related to its clearance from the body. This means that patients with liver or kidney impairment may need lower doses to avoid toxicity. The BNF provides suggested reductions in this situation. This is one reason for using lower doses in elderly patients, but there are other physiological changes with ageing that necessitate lower doses. The starting dose for elderly patients is often half the standard adult dose. Dose titration may be slower and require more careful monitoring in elderly patients.

Bear in mind that plasma concentration is also related to dosing frequency and it may be that manipulating frequency rather than dose is the preferred option (see Chapter 7).

Dose calculations

Dose calculations can be simple or more complex and should always be undertaken with care. It is good practice to ask a colleague to double-check calculations as error is common. Calculations tend to be made on the basis of patient weight or sometimes body surface area. In the case of body weight, doses will generally be expressed as x mg/kg. In addition, weight ranges may be used to match rounded doses (e.g. dalteparin, weight 46–56 kg give 10 000 units). There is usually a maximum dose that should not be exceeded, whatever the weight calculation. If the patient's weight is not known and it cannot be measured in an emergency situation, there is little alternative to guessing, which is often inaccurate. Alternatively, standard weights of 70 kg for a man and 60 kg for a woman are sometimes used.

In pregnancy, the manufacturer often recommends that the dose should be calculated on the basis of the patient's non-pregnant weight. It is important to check this before prescribing.

In some situations using actual body weight in obese patients can result in overdose. Therefore for some medicines with a narrow therapeutic index, such as gentamicin, it is recommended that ideal body weight is used. The formula for calculating ideal body weight is:
- Men 50 kg + 2.3 kg per inch over 5 feet
- Women 45.5 kg + 2.3 kg per inch over 5 feet.

Body surface area calculations are rarely required in adult medicine, except in chemotherapy. Various formulae exist for calculating body surface area based on weight and height measurements, but again patients who are malnourished or obese may be incorrectly dosed. No single formula is recommended (although the BNF uses the DuBois formula), and they are sufficiently complex that it is wise to involve a specialist pharmacist if calculations are needed. Electronic calculation tools are available and may be useful.

The situation is more complex in children (see Chapter 16). In some cases age ranges are used, in others calculations are made based on weight or body surface area. Conflicting information may be available, and in many cases drugs are used off-license and therefore no official dose guidance may exist. The *BNF for Children* should be consulted.

Occasionally, dose estimation by glomerular filtration rate is used, but again you should seek specialist help.

In selected medicines where therapeutic drug monitoring is available, this can be used to adjust doses (see Chapter 21).

9 How to choose route of administration and formulation

Figure 9.1 Different routes of administration.

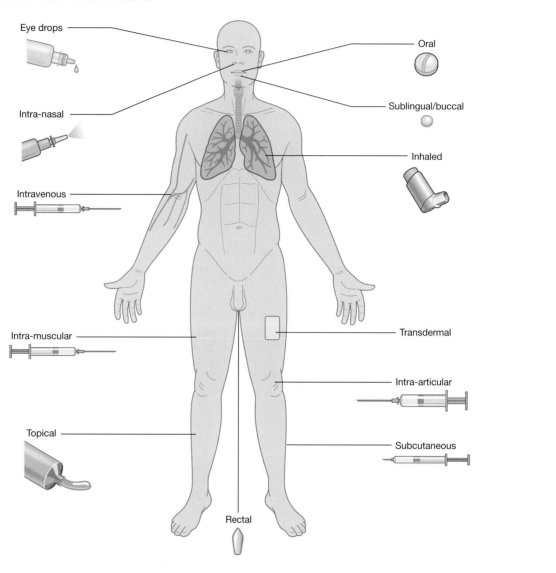

How to choose route of administration

A number of factors should be taken into account when selecting the route of administration that best suits the patient and the goal of treatment. Firstly, what are the available choices (see Figure 9.1)? Many drugs only come in a preparation that is suitable for a single route (usually oral). This may be because there is no particular clinical necessity for other preparations, or because of pharmacokinetic considerations (e.g. insulin, which is a protein, would be digested if taken orally).

Secondly, are there clinical reasons for selecting a particular route? Route of administration should be selected to provide the best efficacy. The intravenous route is most commonly used to ensure a rapid onset of effect or maximum bioavailability. In other instances, a different route may be selected to minimise toxicity (e.g. topical administration or targeting of a particular organ [e.g. lungs targeted with inhalers]). The oral route is preferable in most situations, and in many cases, although intravenous therapy may be ideal, an oral route is a reasonable compromise.

Thirdly, what is practicable for the patient? In some circumstances, the normal or first-choice route may be compromised. In the case of oral medication, issues with nausea and vomiting or swallowing may limit its use. There may be concerns about the patient's ability to self-administer via particular routes (e.g. subcutaneous injections or difficult to use inhalers). The choice may vary if the patient is an inpatient or outpatient, or if the treatment is short term or longer term. If no sensible alternative is possible, patients may need the assistance of a family member, district nurse or other healthcare worker to administer their medication.

Tolerability may also be a consideration. For example, in palliative care it is more usual to give subcutaneous than intramuscular or intravenous injections as it is less painful.

Different routes have different properties, which may also be important. Intramuscular injections tend to have quite variable bioavailability that can be difficult to predict. This makes the route less suitable in many instances.

The *British National Formulary* (BNF) lists each possible route of administration and the available preparations at the end of the drug monograph. Bear in mind that not all preparations may be stocked locally.

How to choose preparation

Choice of preparation may be determined by the route of administration. Alternatively, different options may exist for the same route. This is most commonly seen in the case of oral medicines. A variety of tablets, capsules, liquids and dispersible preparations may be available, and choice can be made around patient choice and convenience. It is worth noting that there may be a financial cost in doing so. Patients with swallowing difficulties may need liquids or soluble drugs. Feeding tubes (e.g. nasogastric or percutaneous endoscopic gastrostomy) can be used to give medicines, but there are a number of issues with this including a lack of licence for many drugs by this route, problems with tubes blocking, and timing of administration in relation to feeds. Take care when crushing or splitting tablets, as this may not be suitable for a number of reasons (the BNF notes whether tablets are scored for splitting). Occasionally, capsules can be opened and the content sprinkled on food. Consult with a pharmacist in these situations.

Prescribers should be aware that different preparations of the same drug may not be equivalent. This is particularly important for a number of drugs such as diltiazem and lithium where you should always specify the brand name. This can be calculated if conversion from one preparation to another is needed (e.g. patient is nil by mouth), but it is wise to involve a pharmacist to assist in making the conversion safely.

Modified release preparations of certain drugs are available. This may be helpful in reducing the frequency with which they are taken and aiding compliance. It is usual to start with the normal dosing regimen and then convert to the modified release preparation, although this is not always necessary.

How to choose duration of treatment, define treatment objectives and measure outcomes

How to choose duration of treatment

When starting a drug, it is important to have in mind the treatment duration. It is easy for a drug to be initiated by a prescriber who will not be involved with the patient's care when it should be discontinued. If the initial decision is not explicit, the patient may be unintentionally over-treated, putting them at risk of adverse effects.

The first general consideration in planning treatment duration is whether this it is a short-term (e.g. a course of antibiotics) or long-term treatment. For many conditions, a short course of medication is appropriate. In the case of antibiotics, a balance should be struck between too short, which may encourage resistance to develop, or too long a duration, which may be unnecessary and put the patient at risk of adverse effects. Local guidance and other sources of information such as the *British National Formulary* (BNF) may quote minimum durations for different infections. Different durations may be recommended for different patient groups (e.g. urinary tract infection in women can usually be managed with 3 days of treatment, but 7 days is suggested for men).

Long-term treatments should also be reviewed after an interval appropriate to the drug and condition in order to evaluate the effect and decide whether to continue the drug. Defining outcomes at the start of treatment makes this easier. Occasionally drugs have a maximum duration that is usually due to safety concerns. If so, it is critical that this is clear to all relevant healthcare workers and to the patient.

How much to dispense at a time

The quantity of medication dispensed may be set by local policy, but may need adjustment in specific cases. It makes sense to only prescribe the quantity needed for a short course of treatment. In long-term conditions, it may not always be appropriate to dispense the normal 1- or 2-month supply usually given. The prescriber should consider the potential risks of overdose, dependence and even selling of treatment. Certain preparations (e.g. eye drops, GTN sprays) can deteriorate over time, becoming ineffective. It would be wasteful to prescribe these in large quantities. It is also worth considering convenience – it may be reasonable to round up to a pack size.

Treatment objectives and outcomes

The objective of treatment, and ways of measuring whether this has been achieved, is important in helping to evaluate whether a treatment is working and when it should be stopped.

There are a number of types of treatment objective. These may be the resolution of symptoms, a change in clinical signs, an objective change in an investigation result, or a particular drug plasma concentration. The resolution or improvement of symptoms is somewhat subjective and may vary from patient to patient. A more objective marker may be desirable. This may be a surrogate such as blood pressure, which would reflect the treatment aim of reducing the risk of stroke. It may be a blood test, such as glycosylated haemoglobin or total cholesterol. It may be the disappearance of X-ray changes or a negative microbiology culture. In the case of anticoagulation, it may be an international normalisation ratio within the target range. You should set out this objective and the timescale within which any examination or investigation should occur.

Prescribers may be limited in what they can reasonably measure. It is likely that the local laboratory will only be able to measure a small range of drug concentrations. The frequency of investigations may also be constrained by cost.

A lack of efficacy does not necessarily mean that a drug should be stopped. It may be that the dose is insufficient, or that the patient is not adhering to treatment correctly. However, if you conclude that treatment is not effective, this is a good time to review the original diagnosis and treatment objective, as well as the drug choice.

When reviewing whether drug therapy is effective, you should also consider its safety. This may be by asking patients about any adverse effects, by checking for signs of organ damage where these are predictable from knowledge of the drug or by checking for toxic plasma concentrations. It is important to schedule these checks when starting a treatment. The BNF gives some guidance about what should be checked (e.g. a full blood count) at what intervals, but you should also be able to predict possible problems from the drug action and possible toxic effects.

Criteria for stopping a drug may be laid down at the outset in some situations. Making this explicit to the patient can also help them to monitor their treatment, and can make it easier to persuade them to stop a drug that is ineffective.

Prescribing at a Glance, First Edition. Sarah Ross. © 2014 John Wiley & Sons, Ltd. Published 2014 by John Wiley & Sons, Ltd.

Companion website: www.ataglanceseries.com/prescribing

11 Assessing suitability of treatment regimens for patients

Does the drug of choice suit this patient?

As described in Chapter 6, when selecting a new drug you should come up with an 'ideal' first-line treatment. The second step is deciding whether that treatment is suitable for the individual patient. The main issues are efficacy and safety. The first-line treatment should be efficacious, but it may be necessary to consider whether this is the case for all patients. Is there anything about this specific patient that would make the treatment less useful? An example of this might be antihypertensive drugs such as angiotensin-converting enzyme inhibitors that are generally less effective in non-white patients.

Next, consider whether there are any reasons why the chosen drug would be less safe in this particular patient. Is there a history of allergy to this or related drugs (e.g. patients who are allergic to penicillins may also react to carbapenems and cephalosporins)? Bear in mind contraindications caused by renal or hepatic impairment or special circumstances such as pregnancy. Are there any other diseases that the patient has which would make the treatment unsuitable? For example, a beta-blocker would be contraindicated in a patient with asthma.

Next consider any drug–drug interactions that will occur if the new drug is added to the patient's existing medicines. Not all interactions are necessarily problematic (see Chapter 23).

If the first-choice drug is unsuitable, what alternative treatment is the next best option? In some instances, this may be a different drug from the same class (e.g. one calcium channel blocker may be implicated in a drug–drug interaction where another is not), but in others it may mean the drug class is contraindicated. This may require reconsideration of the safety and efficacy of all other possible treatments, or the prescriber may have a second choice ready for such situations.

Is the standard dose regimen suitable?

Once you are sure that the drug is suitable, consider whether any alteration to the standard regimen is needed in order to ensure the drug is safe and effective. Does the patient have any condition that may cause changes in the patient's capacity to absorb, distribute, metabolise or excrete the drug, or cause changes in sensitivity to the drug? This may be because of co-existing disease or to age. Elderly patients, for example, are often more sensitive to drug effects while having reduced capacity to metabolise and excrete drugs. They may need a reduced plasma concentration, which can be achieved by reducing either the dose or frequency of administration. In general, reducing the dose is a simple and effective action.

In some patients, an increased plasma concentration will be needed in order to have an effect. In general, increasing the frequency is safer than increasing the dose (fewer peaks and troughs).

It is also sensible to consider whether the regimen is convenient for the individual patient. Some patients may be less able to remember a regimen that requires several doses a day. It may be worth considering a different drug or regimen if compliance is likely to be poor.

Similarly, the prescriber should think about whether the standard duration of treatment is suitable. The prescription should provide sufficient drug to treat the indication, without giving so much that there is waste or the possibility of addiction or abuse.

Prescribing at a Glance, First Edition. Sarah Ross. © 2014 John Wiley & Sons, Ltd. Published 2014 by John Wiley & Sons, Ltd.
Companion website: www.ataglanceseries.com/prescribing

12 Worked example 1: Chapters 6–11

Figure 12.1

A 35-year-old man attends the Accident and Emergency (A&E) department complaining of a swollen, painful left ankle following a game of football. A simple sprain is diagnosed and he is discharged with analgesia.

What would be appropriate analgesia?

Step 1   Define the treatment goal

The aim of treatment in this situation is pain relief and reduction of inflammation.

Step 2   Compare drug classes for ideal treatment

A list like this can be created:

- Paracetamol
- Non-steroidal anti-inflammatories (NSAIDs)
- Weak opioids
- Strong opioids.

Next, compare these on safety, efficacy, general suitability and cost for this indication to produce a table like this:

Drug class	Safety	Efficacy	Suitability	Cost
Paracetamol	+++	++	++++	++++
NSAIDs	++	+++	++	++++
Weak opioids	+++	+ (better in combination)	++++	++++
Strong opioids	++	++	+++	++ to ++++

From this, the ideal drug class would be NSAIDs as these have anti-inflammatory action as well as analgesic effect. Another way of looking at this would be to consult a guideline such as the WHO pain ladder. This would support starting with paracetamol, but also allows for suitable adjuncts such as NSAIDs where appropriate.

The best option might be paracetamol and an NSAID.

Step 3   Compare individual drugs in chosen class

A wide range of NSAIDs are available; however, in any one A&E department, there are likely to be a smaller range to choose from.

A similar table can be constructed to compare individual drugs. This table might reflect the availability of NSAIDs within one particular hospital:

Based on this analysis, naproxen would be a good choice.

Drug	Safety	Efficacy	Suitability	Cost
Ibuprofen	+++	++	++	++++
Diclofenac	++	+++	++	++++
Naproxen	+++	+++	++	++++
Celecoxib	+++	+++	++	+

Step 4   Suitability of chosen drug for patient

- Is there anything about this choice of paracetamol and naproxen that is unsuitable for the patient?
- Contraindications would include a history of asthma, renal impairment or gastrointestinal bleeding. Other issues include heart disease or hypertension, allergy to NSAIDs or bleeding disorders.
- If the patient was pregnant, breast feeding, elderly or very young, these would also need to be taken into consideration.
  None of these should be a problem.

Step 5   Choose dose, frequency, route

- An oral route is usually best if the drug is available in a suitable formulation and if the patient is able to take it. There is no indication in this case to use any other route.
- The standard dose of paracetamol is 1 g (unless the patient is under 50 kg).
- The BNF states that the dose of naproxen should be 500 mg for the first dose and 250 mg 6- to 8-hourly as required. It is usually sensible to start treatment at the lower end of any range.
- It would be reasonable to suggest regular dosing in the first few days to maximize the benefits of the treatment.
  The prescription could be for:
    – Paracetamol 1 g four times a day for 1 week
    – Naproxen 250 mg three times a day for 1 week

Step 6   Monitor effects

- The main method of monitoring whether the treatment is working is to ask the patient about pain and swelling of the ankle. It is unlikely that a routine appointment will be needed, so the patient should be asked to attend his GP if the pain does not settle and more than 1 week of treatment is needed.
- The patient should be warned about likely side effects, in this case gastrointestinal upset.
- As treatment is for a short course only, other monitoring is not needed in this patient who is at low risk of serious adverse effects.

Prescribing at a Glance, First Edition. Sarah Ross. © 2014 John Wiley & Sons, Ltd. Published 2014 by John Wiley & Sons, Ltd.
Companion website: www.ataglanceseries.com/prescribing

13 Worked example 2: Chapters 6–11

Figure 13.1

A 55-year-old man is admitted to hospital complaining of breathlessness and right-sided pleuritic chest pain following a knee operation 1 week ago. Pulmonary embolism is diagnosed.

What would be the most appropriate *initial* treatment?

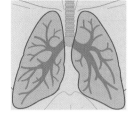

Step 1 Define the treatment goal

The aim of treatment in this situation is to prevent further venous thromboembolism in the *next few days*.

Step 2 Compare drug classes for ideal treatment

A list like this can be created:

- unfractionated heparin
- low molecular weight heparin (LMWH)
- warfarin
- fondaparinux
- new oral anticoagulants (e.g. dabigatran).

These judgements relate to short-term use, and considerations would be different for longer term use where an oral option would be desirable. From this analysis, the ideal drug class would be LMWHs given their quick onset of action, good safety profile, greater convenience than unfractionated heparin and relatively low cost. Remember that choosing a medicine you are familiar with using is also important.

In real life, your choice may be directed by a hospital policy and formulary

Next, compare these on safety, efficacy, general suitability and cost for this indication to produce a table like this:

Drug class	Safety	Efficacy	Suitability	Cost
Unfractionated heparin	+++ (can be stopped quickly; narrow therapeutic index)	++++	++ (intravenous infusion less convenient)	++++
Low molecular weight heparin	++++ (partial antidote)	++++	+++ (subcutaneous injection)	+++
Warfarin	+++ (narrow therapeutic index; wide inter-patient variability)	++ (may take up to 48 hours to work)	++ (oral)	++++
Fondaparinux	+++ (no antidote)	++++	+++ (subcutaneous injection)	+++
New oral anticoagulants	+++ (new, so less well known; no antidote available; may be safer than warfarin)	++++	+++	+

Step 3 Compare individual drugs in chosen class

Several LMWHs are available; however, in any one hospital there is likely to be only one or perhaps two available.

A similar table can be constructed to compare individual drugs: however there are no important differences recognised between low molecular weight heparins.

Based on this analysis, any one of dalteparin, enoxaparin and tinzaparin would be a good choice. This example will use dalteparin.

Step 4 Suitability of chosen drug for patient

Is there anything about this patient that would make this choice unsuitable?

None of these should be problematic for this patient.

Step 5 Choose dose, frequency, route

There is only one available route for dalteparin, the subcutaneous route.

The dose is based on patient weight (and rounded to the next suitable pre-filled syringe). The standard 70 kg man would require 15 000 units once a day according to the *British National Formulary*.

Step 6 Monitor effects

The main way of monitoring whether the treatment is working is to monitor for further signs of embolism.

The patient should be warned about likely side effects, in this case bruising and bleeding.

As treatment is for a short course only, other monitoring is not needed in this patient who is at low risk of serious adverse effects. Monitoring the platelet count and potassium level is recommended if heparin is used for more than a few days.

Prescribing at a Glance, First Edition. Sarah Ross. © 2014 John Wiley & Sons, Ltd. Published 2014 by John Wiley & Sons, Ltd.
Companion website: www.ataglanceseries.com/prescribing

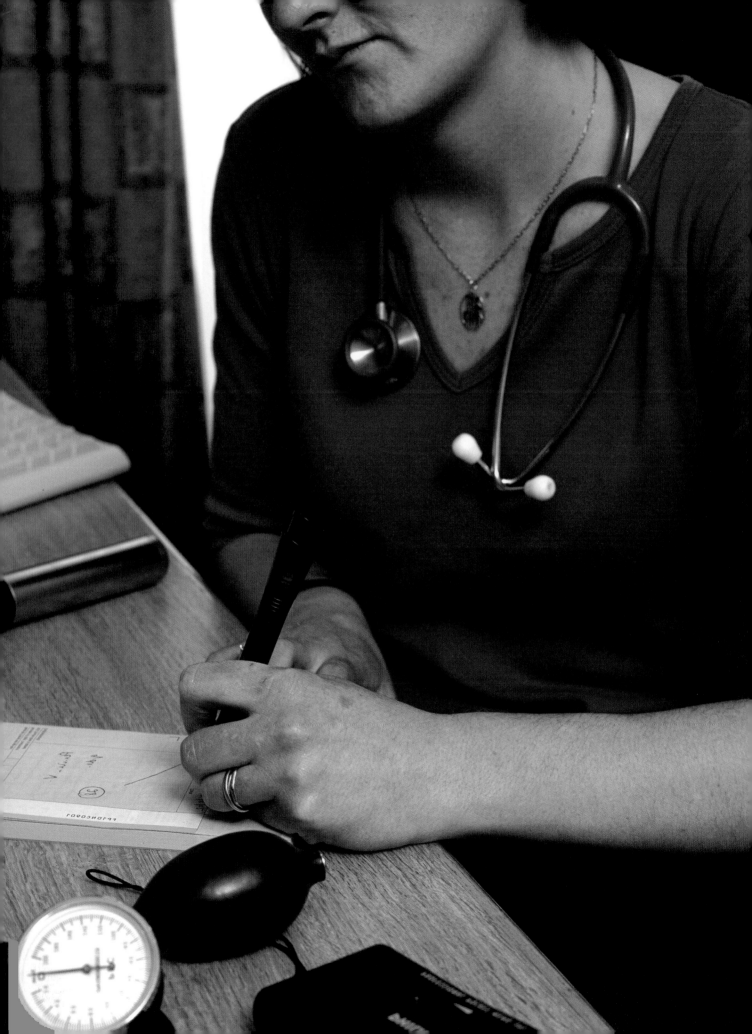

Prescribing for special groups

Part 3

Chapters

 Don't forget to visit the companion website for this book
www.ataglanceseries.com/prescribing to do some
practice MCQs and case studies on these topics.

Prescribing in liver disease

Figure 14.1 Pharmacokinetic changes in liver disease.

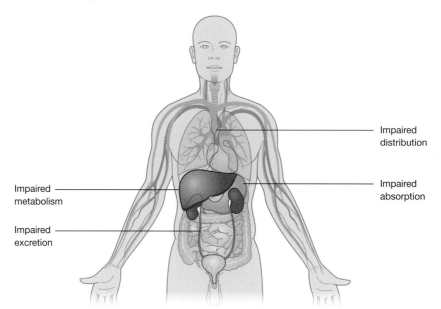

Impaired distribution

Impaired absorption

Impaired metabolism

Impaired excretion

Table 14.1 Child-Pugh classification

Score	1	2	3
Bilirubin (micromol/L)	<34	34–50	>50
Albumin (g/L)	>35	28–35	<28
International normalised ratio	<1.7	1.7–2.0	>2.0
Ascites	–	+	++
Encephalopathy	–	+	++

If the patient has either primary biliary cirrhosis or sclerosing cholangitis, bilirubin levels are redefined as <68 micromol/L = 1; 68-170 micromol/L = 2; >170 micromol/L = 3.
The individual scores are then summed and classified as follows:
• 4-6 = A
• 7-9 = B
• 10-15 = C
Adapted from: Pugh RNH, Murray-Lyon IM, Dawson JL et al.
Transection of the oesophagus for bleeding oesophageal varices. *Br J Surg* 1973;**60**:649-9.

What is different about patients with liver disease?

The liver is the major organ involved in metabolism of drugs, and any reduction in its capacity to do so can be problematic. In addition, a number of other pharmacokinetic and pharmacodynamic processes can be affected by liver disease. Consequently, some drugs are contraindicated or may require dose adjustment. The main changes are noted below (Figure 14.1).

Impaired absorption

Reduced bioavailability of lipid soluble drugs may be seen in cholestasis.

Impaired drug distribution

Hypoalbuminaemia is a feature of severe liver disease, reducing the amount of albumin available for drug binding and increasing the unbound drug concentration. Toxicity may occur in highly protein bound drugs with a narrow therapeutic index (e.g. phenytoin).

Impaired metabolism

Liver disease may reduce the capacity to metabolise certain drugs leading to toxicity. This is caused by both the reduction in the metabolic capacity of the liver and the changes in liver blood flow that can occur. Problems are generally limited to patients with severe liver disease, as the liver has considerable reserve. Estimating liver impairment can be challenging and predicting exactly what will happen in individuals is not always possible. Drugs that have a high hepatic extraction ratio (high first pass metabolism) are particularly problematic.

Impaired excretion

Hepatobiliary disease may lead to drug toxicity if the biliary system is obstructed, as this is a route of excretion for some medicines. Renal impairment can also occur as a consequence of liver disease, and a reduction in glomerular filtration rate may be important for renally cleared drugs.

Altered pharmacodynamics

Common issues with liver disease such as hepatic encephalopathy, ascites and deficiencies in clotting factors can increase sensitivity to particular drug effects. Drugs that cause sedation, constipation or hypokalaemia are contraindicated in severe liver disease as these can cause encephalopathy. Ascites may be worsened by any drug that causes fluid retention (e.g. non-steroidal anti-inflammatory drugs [NSAIDS]). Anticoagulants will require careful monitoring and adjustment, if not complete avoidance, in severe liver disease as clotting factors are usually depleted.

Hepatotoxicity

Many medicines can cause liver damage, through a wide range of mechanisms including: hepatitis, cholestasis, non-alcoholic steatohepatitis and cirrhosis. In theory, these should be avoided wherever possible in patients with liver disease to prevent further hepatic impairment. However, it has been argued that in practice most medications can be used safely in patients with chronic hepatic impairment. In addition, for most drugs, patients with liver disease do not seem to be more susceptible to hepatic injury than the general population. Important exceptions include methotrexate in patients with alcoholic liver disease, and anti-tuberculous drugs and anti-human immunodeficiency virus drugs in patients with hepatitis B or C.

Selecting medicines and regimens in liver disease

As with all medicines, it is important to consider the risks and benefits of treatment in each individual patient. The following principles may be useful in weighing these up.

Unlike in renal impairment, there is no well-accepted method of judging the degree of liver impairment when making prescribing decisions. The Child–Pugh (Table 14.1) and Model for End-stage Liver Disease (MELD) classifications may be useful in estimating hepatic metabolic capacity, but they are only a guide. Patients scoring in the B or C range of the Child–Pugh classification (moderate or severe disease) should be regarded as having hepatic impairment. If possible, hepatotoxic drugs should be avoided in these patients; however, this is dependent on the availability of alternative drugs and the strength of the indication for treatment. Similarly, drugs that may worsen the patient's clinical condition (described above) should be avoided.

For drugs that are extensively hepatically metabolised, it may be helpful to consider the drug in terms of whether it has a narrow or wide therapeutic index (i.e. the difference between the effective and toxic doses). If the drug has a narrow therapeutic index, avoid or use with extreme caution. If the therapeutic index is wide, then it may be possible to use the drug with a reduced dose or frequency of administration. Bear in mind that even medicines that are only partially metabolised in the liver may become toxic at normal doses in severe liver disease.

It is also important to consider what type of liver disease the patient has. Cholestatic disease is likely to cause problems with absorption and with biliary excretion of drugs, whereas hepatocellular disease is likely to lead to issues with metabolism.

Drugs that can cause renal impairment should also be used with care in liver disease because of the danger of hepatorenal syndrome.

The *British National Formulary* gives specific information on contraindications and dose adjustments in liver disease.

Specific medicines

Common drugs that require particular care include:
- Paracetamol: need not be completely avoided but lower doses are recommended, including for patients with alcohol excess who do not have proven alcoholic liver disease.
- Aspirin and NSAIDs: the risk of bleeding is increased because of the reduction in clotting factors; in addition, NSAIDs can increase ascites.
- Anticoagulants: the effect of warfarin may be increased because of a reduction in clotting factors. It is likely that thrombin inhibitors will have an increased bleeding risk in liver disease for similar reasons.
- Antidiabetic drugs: there is an increased risk of lactic acidosis with metformin therapy. An increased risk of hypoglycaemia is seen with sulphonylureas. Glitazones should be avoided because of the potential for hepatotoxicity.
- Opiates and benzodiazepines: their use may precipitate encephalopathy, and are best avoided in severe liver disease.

15 Prescribing in renal disease

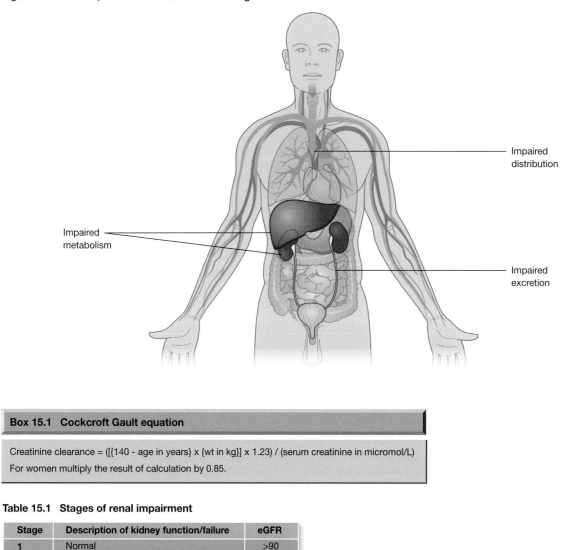

Figure 15.1 The impact of renal disease on dosing.

Impaired distribution

Impaired metabolism

Impaired excretion

Box 15.1 Cockcroft Gault equation

Creatinine clearance = ([{140 - age in years} x {wt in kg}] x 1.23) / (serum creatinine in micromol/L)
For women multiply the result of calculation by 0.85.

Table 15.1 Stages of renal impairment

Stage	Description of kidney function/failure	eGFR
1	Normal	>90
2	Mild	60–89
3	Moderate	30–59
4	Severe	15–29
5	Established	<15

eGFR, estimated glomerular filtration rate.

Prescribing at a Glance, First Edition. Sarah Ross. © 2014 John Wiley & Sons, Ltd. Published 2014 by John Wiley & Sons, Ltd.
Companion website: www.ataglanceseries.com/prescribing

What is different about patients with renal disease?

The kidney is the major organ involved in excretion of drugs. Although there is a degree of redundancy, any decrease in glomerular filtration rate (GFR) is potentially problematic in terms of effective drug clearance. In addition, other pharmacokinetic and pharmacodynamic changes can occur in renal disease, which may impact dosing (Figure 15.1).

Impaired distribution

Protein binding may be altered either because of hypoalbuminaemia (caused by proteinuria) or uraemia. Reductions in protein binding capacity can lead to toxicity in highly protein bound drugs with a narrow therapeutic index.

Impaired metabolism

Certain drugs are metabolised in the kidney and may be affected by various types of renal disease. In addition, liver metabolism of drugs tends to be slower in chronic renal disease.

Impaired excretion

The kidney excretes drugs through the processes of glomerular filtration, active tubular secretion and resorption. All these functions are reduced in renal disease. Drugs that are renally cleared may require dose adjustment or avoidance.

Pharmacodynamic changes

Increased sensitivity to various drug adverse effects can be seen.

Nephrotoxicity

Many commonly used drugs are nephrotoxic at pre-renal, intrinsic or post-renal levels. Dehydration or reduced renal perfusion are pre-renal causes. Many drugs cause intrinsic renal damage by acute tubular necrosis or acute interstitial nephritis. Post-renal obstruction can be occasionally drug induced. Nephrotoxic drugs should be avoided if possible in patients with renal disease as they may cause further reduction in renal function.

Selecting medicines and regimes in renal disease

The following principles may be useful in weighing up the risks and benefits in renal patients.

Classification of renal function is important, and is normally approximated by the GFR. Creatinine levels alone are a poor indicator of GFR, particularly in the elderly where a reduction in muscle mass may lead to a lower creatinine level. There are a number of ways of estimating the GFR using creatinine clearance (Cockcroft Gault equation, Box 15.1) or the estimated GFR (eGFR), which is now calculated by many laboratories. These are not interchangeable, and prescribing guidance has generally been based on GFR as defined by creatinine clearance. The *British National Formulary* (BNF) now uses eGFR, but recommends reverting to the Cockcroft Gault formula for toxic drugs with a narrow safety margin or when dealing with extremes in weight.

Renal impairment is classified as shown in Table 15.1. Specific guidance for individual drugs is provided using these categories. It is important to use up-to-date blood tests when prescribing.

Where possible, nephrotoxic drugs should be avoided and the total number of drugs kept to a minimum. Ideally, choose agents that do not require renal metabolism to an active form or renal excretion (of the drug or its active metabolites). Close monitoring is required to check for any deterioration in renal function following the addition of a new medicine.

If there is no obvious alternative to a renally cleared drug, consider its therapeutic index. If the drug has a narrow therapeutic index, avoid or use it with extreme caution. If the therapeutic index is wide, then it may be possible to use the drug with a reduced dose or frequency of administration. BNF guidance is available; information may also be found in the Schedule of Product Characteristics and in *The Renal Handbook*. Remember that these sources may not be consistent. It is important to realise that these are only guides, and that individual patients may differ. Therapeutic drug monitoring may be needed to guide dosing. While caution is essential, it is also important not to undertreat patients with renal impairment. Specialist help will be invaluable.

For patients on dialysis, there are further considerations. New prescribers should not tackle these patients alone, but should be guided by specialist medical and pharmacy colleagues.

Loading doses may be needed in renal impairment as time to steady-state concentration is related to the half-life of the drug. This half-life is prolonged by reduced clearance, and so the time to steady state is longer. A loading dose may be needed to achieve the desired effect in a timely manner.

Specific medicines

Nephrotoxins

The following commonly used drugs should be avoided where possible in renal impairment:

• Antibiotics: aminoglycosides are highly nephrotoxic, but on occasion may be required. Close monitoring of renal function and of drug concentration is needed to reduce the risk of toxicity. Other antibiotics may need dose reduction.
• Non-steroidal anti-inflammatory drugs (NSAIDs): all NSAIDs and COX-2 inhibitors affect renal prostaglandins and can cause renal damage. This is more likely in patients who are hypovolaemic, using angiotensin-converting-enzyme (ACE) inhibitors/angiotensin receptor blockers (ARBs) or with pre-existing renal disease.
• ACE inhibitors and ARB: these drugs can be useful in preserving renal function in diabetes and may be beneficial in reducing renal damage from hypertension. However, they can also cause significant nephrotoxicity, particularly in renal artery stenosis. Senior advice is needed before initiating.
• Diuretics: thiazide diuretics are ineffective if GFR <30. Loop diuretics may be needed in renal disease, but can also induce hypovolaemia which can be damaging.

Renally cleared drugs

Drugs that are renally cleared and may require dose adjustments to limit toxicity include insulins and other antidiabetic medicines, digoxin and aminoglycosides. Opioids that are renally metabolised may require dose adjustment or use of an alternative.

Drugs in renal transplantation

Immunosuppressant therapy is needed in transplant patients to reduce the risk of rejection. Azathioprine, mycophenolate mofetil, calcineurin inhibitors (e.g. ciclosporin, tacrolimus) and basiliximab are commonly used. More information is given on these drugs in Chapter 35. Withholding or stopping these drugs can cause transplant rejection and therefore they should not be stopped without consultation with the patient's usual medical team.

16 Prescribing in children

Figure 16.1 Page from the *British National Formulary for Children*.
(Source: Joint Formulary Committee 2013, p. 45. Reproduced with permission from the British Medical Association and Royal Pharmaceutical Society of Great Britain.)

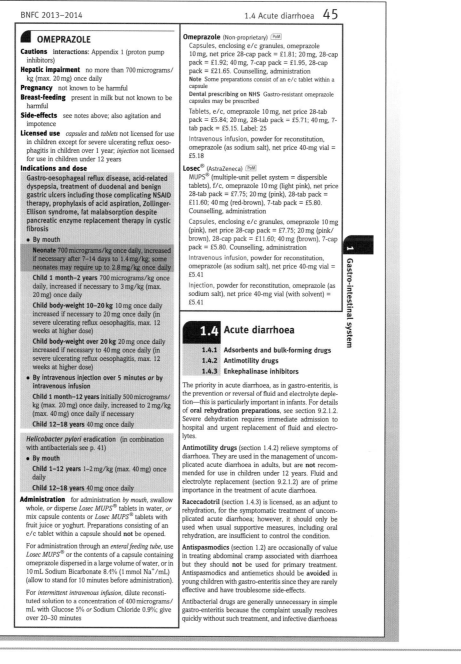

BNFC 2013–2014   1.4 Acute diarrhoea   45

OMEPRAZOLE

Cautions interactions: Appendix 1 (proton pump inhibitors)

Hepatic impairment no more than 700 micrograms/kg (max. 20 mg) once daily

Pregnancy not known to be harmful

Breast-feeding present in milk but not known to be harmful

Side-effects see notes above; also agitation and impotence

Licensed use *capsules* and *tablets* not licensed for use in children except for severe ulcerating reflux oeso-phagitis in children over 1 year; *injection* not licensed for use in children under 12 years

Indications and dose

Gastro-oesophageal reflux disease, acid-related dyspepsia, treatment of duodenal and benign gastric ulcers including those complicating NSAID therapy, prophylaxis of acid aspiration, Zollinger-Ellison syndrome, fat malabsorption despite pancreatic enzyme replacement therapy in cystic fibrosis

- **By mouth**

  Neonate 700 micrograms/kg once daily, increased if necessary after 7–14 days to 1.4 mg/kg; some neonates may require up to 2.8 mg/kg once daily

  Child 1 month–2 years 700 micrograms/kg once daily, increased if necessary to 3 mg/kg (max. 20 mg) once daily

  Child body-weight 10–20 kg 10 mg once daily increased if necessary to 20 mg once daily (in severe ulcerating reflux oesophagitis, max. 12 weeks at higher dose)

  Child body-weight over 20 kg 20 mg once daily increased if necessary to 40 mg once daily (in severe ulcerating reflux oesophagitis, max. 12 weeks at higher dose)

- **By intravenous injection over 5 minutes *or* by intravenous infusion**

  Child 1 month–12 years initially 500 micrograms/kg (max. 20 mg) once daily, increased to 2 mg/kg (max. 40 mg) once daily if necessary

  Child 12–18 years 40 mg once daily

Helicobacter pylori eradication (in combination with antibacterials see p. 41)

- **By mouth**

  Child 1–12 years 1–2 mg/kg (max. 40 mg) once daily

  Child 12–18 years 40 mg once daily

Administration for administration *by mouth*, swallow whole, *or* disperse *Losec MUPS®* tablets in water, *or* mix capsule contents or *Losec MUPS®* tablets with fruit juice or yoghurt. Preparations consisting of an e/c tablet within a capsule should **not** be opened.

For administration through an *enteral feeding tube*, use *Losec MUPS®* or the contents of a capsule containing omeprazole dispersed in a large volume of water, or in 10 mL Sodium Bicarbonate 8.4% (1 mmol Na⁺/mL) (allow to stand for 10 minutes before administration).

For *intermittent intravenous infusion*, dilute reconstituted solution to a concentration of 400 micrograms/mL with Glucose 5% *or* Sodium Chloride 0.9%; give over 20–30 minutes

Omeprazole (Non-proprietary) [PoM]
Capsules, enclosing e/c granules, omeprazole 10 mg, net price 28-cap pack = £1.81; 20 mg, 28-cap pack = £1.92; 40 mg, 7-cap pack = £1.95, 28-cap pack = £21.65. Counselling, administration
Note Some preparations consist of an e/c tablet within a capsule
Dental prescribing on NHS Gastro-resistant omeprazole capsules may be prescribed

Tablets, e/c, omeprazole 10 mg, net price 28-tab pack = £5.84; 20 mg, 28-tab pack = £5.71; 40 mg, 7-tab pack = £5.15. Label: 25

Intravenous infusion, powder for reconstitution, omeprazole (as sodium salt), net price 40-mg vial = £5.18

Losec® (AstraZeneca) [PoM]
MUPS® (multiple-unit pellet system = dispersible tablets), f/c, omeprazole 10 mg (light pink), net price 28-tab pack = £7.75; 20 mg (pink), 28-tab pack = £11.60; 40 mg (red-brown), 7-tab pack = £5.80. Counselling, administration

Capsules, enclosing e/c granules, omeprazole 10 mg (pink), net price 28-cap pack = £7.75; 20 mg (pink/brown), 28-cap pack = £11.60; 40 mg (brown), 7-cap pack = £5.80. Counselling, administration

Intravenous infusion, powder for reconstitution, omeprazole (as sodium salt), net price 40-mg vial = £5.41

Injection, powder for reconstitution, omeprazole (as sodium salt), net price 40-mg vial (with solvent) = £5.41

1.4 Acute diarrhoea

1.4.1 Adsorbents and bulk-forming drugs
1.4.2 Antimotility drugs
1.4.3 Enkephalinase inhibitors

The priority in acute diarrhoea, as in gastro-enteritis, is the prevention or reversal of fluid and electrolyte depletion—this is particularly important in infants. For details of **oral rehydration preparations**, see section 9.2.1.2. Severe dehydration requires immediate admission to hospital and urgent replacement of fluid and electrolytes.

Antimotility drugs (section 1.4.2) relieve symptoms of diarrhoea. They are used in the management of uncomplicated acute diarrhoea in adults, but are **not** recommended for use in children under 12 years. Fluid and electrolyte replacement (section 9.2.1.2) are of prime importance in the treatment of acute diarrhoea.

Racecadotril (section 1.4.3) is licensed, as an adjunct to rehydration, for the symptomatic treatment of uncomplicated acute diarrhoea; however, it should only be used when usual supportive measures, including oral rehydration, are insufficient to control the condition.

Antispasmodics (section 1.2) are occasionally of value in treating abdominal cramp associated with diarrhoea but they should **not** be used for primary treatment. Antispasmodics and antiemetics should be **avoided** in young children with gastro-enteritis since they are rarely effective and have troublesome side-effects.

Antibacterial drugs are generally unnecessary in simple gastro-enteritis because the complaint usually resolves quickly without such treatment, and infective diarrhoeas

1

Gastro-intestinal system

Prescribing at a Glance, First Edition. Sarah Ross. © 2014 John Wiley & Sons, Ltd. Published 2014 by John Wiley & Sons, Ltd.
Companion website: www.ataglanceseries.com/prescribing

What is different about children

Prescribing for children is more complex than prescribing for adults for a number of reasons. Firstly, pharmacokinetics and pharmacodynamics are different in children, and they also vary between different age groups. Secondly, clinical trials are rarely conducted in children, meaning that there is little data available for many drugs leading to 'off-label' or 'off-license' use. Thirdly, there may be issues around compliance and route of administration. Finally, medication errors can occur more easily as many prescriptions will require calculations to be made, and any errors in calculation can be more serious than in adults. On the positive side, children are less likely than adults to be subject to polypharmacy.

Pharmacokinetic changes

Drug absorption is similar to adults, although gut transit time and gastric acid levels vary with age. Distribution can be quite different, as body composition is altered (increased total body water in neonate that decreases with age) and reduced plasma protein levels. Different enzyme systems mature at different rates, but overall metabolism is lower in neonates, rising to adult levels in the first few months and then exceeding adult rates for the majority of childhood. Renal clearance is reduced in the neonate, and the kidneys reach maturity at about 6 months of age. Excretion rates may be higher in children than in adults.

Licensing issues

As a result of the difficulties inherent in testing medicines in children, data can be scarce and a license may only cover adult use. 'Off-label' use, where the medicine is used in an age group different from the license, is relatively common in children. 'Off-license' treatment may occur where a licensed product is reformulated for children. The use of such medicines may be unavoidable, but adverse drug reactions (ADRs) are a risk without adequate safety data. Because of the differences between children and adults, these ADRs may be different to those in adults and can be more challenging to identify, particularly in young children. In recent years, progress has been made as efforts have been made to gather what data does exist in publications such as the *British National Formulary for Children* (BNFC) (Figure 16.1).

Compliance

Greater consideration of the route of administration may be needed in children, bearing in mind that the taste may be unpleasant or administration difficult. The child's ability to use inhalers or other devices should be considered. A spacer may be needed. It is usually helpful to minimise the frequency of administration and the total number of drugs. It is also important that parents understand the reasons for medication, as they may be concerned about side effects. In older children, peer pressure may influence willingness to use medicines.

Selecting medicines and regimens in children

Similar principles apply to selecting medicines for children as do for adults, but it is even more important to be sure that drug therapy is needed.

Dosage should be checked with a paediatric reference, such as the BNFC, although local protocols may be available. As doses are often calculated by weight within an age bracket, a measure of accurate weight is critical. Be aware of the possibility of calculation errors; it is good practice to obtain a double check on calculations. In hospital situations it is wise to seek the assistance of a paediatric pharmacist or senior member of the team. Doses may need to be rounded depending on the administration method. Where this happens, round down.

Try to keep the frequency of dosing to a minimum and reduce the total number of medicines. This may be achieved by selecting one drug rather than another from the same class (e.g. clarithromycin [twice a day] versus erythromycin [four times a day]). Timing of doses can be varied around the child's regime, rather than sticking rigidly to dose schedules.

Care should be taken over the preparation used. Oral administration is normally preferable, but consideration should be given as to how this will be achieved. Oral syringes may be helpful for liquid preparations, both in ensuring accurate measuring and also easier administration.

Parents should be advised not to mix oral medicines with infant feed. Some tablets may be crushed, but not all, so it is important that parents are given appropriate instructions. Sugar-free preparations should be used to reduce the risk of dental caries.

Other routes can be used, especially in unwell children where the oral route is often unreliable. Rectal administration may be appropriate, but bear in mind that absorption is more erratic, which can be problematic with certain drugs. Intramuscular injection may not be suitable because of low muscle mass. It is also very painful, so is typically only used for vaccination. The intravenous route is more challenging in children than in adults and other options may have to be found. It is important, however, that in acute situations the need for treatment of the child should outweigh any reluctance to use particular routes.

Where to find information about medicines in children

The Schedule of Product Characteristics may be helpful, but in many cases the lack of data will lead manufacturers to state that the drug is not suitable for children. More practical information is given in the BNFC, which gives guidance on licensing, suitability for children, dosage guidance by indication and by age group (note age grouping may be different for different drugs), and on administration.

17 Prescribing in the elderly

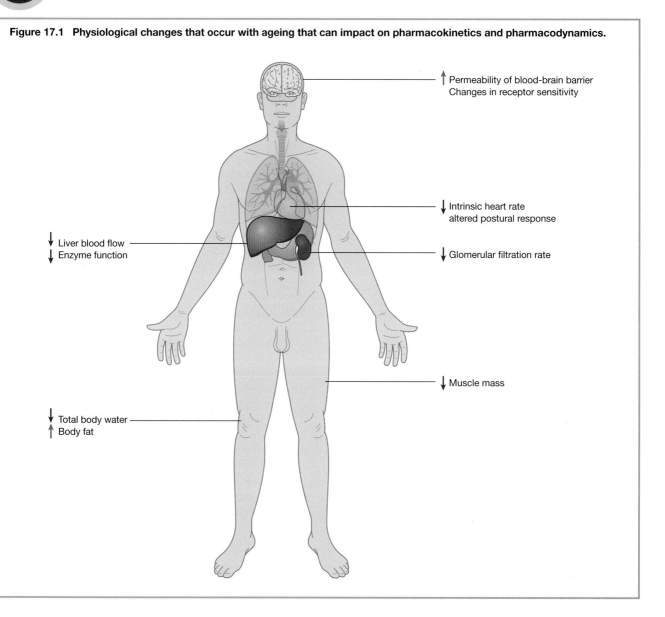

Figure 17.1 Physiological changes that occur with ageing that can impact on pharmacokinetics and pharmacodynamics.

↑ Permeability of blood-brain barrier
Changes in receptor sensitivity

↓ Liver blood flow
↓ Enzyme function

↓ Intrinsic heart rate
altered postural response

↓ Glomerular filtration rate

↓ Muscle mass

↓ Total body water
↑ Body fat

What is different about elderly patients?

In most areas of medicine, a significant proportion of patients are elderly. Physiological changes caused by ageing can be important in pharmacokinetics and pharmacodynamics (Figure 17.1). This varies between patients but should be considered before prescribing.

Drug absorption rates may be reduced by ageing, with a longer time needed to reach peak concentrations, but overall absorption levels are similar. First pass metabolism, by which drugs are absorbed and then metabolised in the liver before reaching the systemic circulation, can be reduced because of decreased liver mass and blood flow. This means that drugs that would normally undergo significant initial metabolism have higher plasma concen-

trations. This can also affect pro-drugs (which require metabolism to change from an inactive to active form), which will have lower bioavailability.

Drug distribution can be affected by the changes in body composition (i.e. proportionally less muscle mass and total body water; more body fat). This can affect the volume of distribution, which may result in either increased plasma concentrations or half-life of the drug, causing toxicity. Although in theory protein binding may also be changed, this seems to have little noticeable clinical effect.

Drug metabolism can be reduced by loss of hepatic enzymes, which may mean increases in plasma concentrations.

Drug excretion can be reduced as a result of the decrease in glomerular filtration rate (GFR) seen with ageing (at least 50% reduction in GFR by age 70).

Prescribing at a Glance, First Edition. Sarah Ross. © 2014 John Wiley & Sons, Ltd. Published 2014 by John Wiley & Sons, Ltd.
Companion website: www.ataglanceseries.com/prescribing

Adverse drug reactions (ADRs) are more common in the elderly as a result of ageing, but also because of increased sensitivity to drug actions and comorbidities. The majority of these ADRs are type A (i.e. predictable and dose related; see Chapter 22). Elderly patients often take multiple medicines, and synergistic adverse effects are seen. Polypharmacy also increases the chance of drug–drug interactions, where again elderly patients may be more vulnerable to unwanted effects.

All these factors contribute to significant medication-induced morbidity and mortality in the elderly.

Selecting medicines and regimens in the elderly

When prescribing in the elderly, consider the following:
• What is the problem you are treating? Is this a symptom or a disease? Where possible, be clear about the diagnosis. Take care not to prescribe a drug to manage an adverse effect from another treatment unless this is unavoidable.
• Consider whether drug therapy is the best therapeutic action, or whether a non-pharmacological approach might be better.
• Think about whether the drug you are considering using causes particular problems in elderly patients or has a narrow safety margin (e.g. warfarin). Can it be safely used in this patient?
• Check in the *British National Formulary* to see whether a lower dose is recommended in the elderly. Start with the lowest dose and titrate up slowly.
• Review the new drug soon and check whether it is achieving your aim. Review all prescriptions regularly and stop any medicines that are not beneficial.
• Try to keep the drug regimens as simple as possible. Consider compliance issues that elderly patients in particular may experience (e.g. forgetfulness, difficulty opening packaging).
Elderly patients should not be denied proven beneficial medicines on the basis of age, but bear in mind that clinical trials are often performed in a younger population, which may mean that benefits do not translate to an older age group.

Specific medicines

Some drugs are more challenging to use in elderly patients, and some are best avoided altogether.

Hypnotics

Benzodiazepines should not be routinely prescribed for insomnia, but often are. Increased sensitivity to benzodiazepines is well recognised with increasing age, as is a possible increase in half-life, both of which contribute to 'hangover' effects seen the next day. Patients are at increased risk of falls and cognitive impairment. If a benzodiazepine must be used, choose one with a short half-life such as lorazepam and use for the shortest possible time.

Neuroleptic drugs, often prescribed for agitation in the elderly, can cause delirium, extrapyramidal symptoms and postural hypotension in the short term and possibly stroke in the longer term. Again, avoid these if possible and consider other non-pharmacological measures.

Analgesics

Opioid sensitivity is increased in the elderly as is a reduction in clearance. Starting doses of 25% to 50% of normal adult doses are recommended in the elderly. Tramadol works on serotonin and adrenergic receptors as well as opioid ones, giving it a different side-effect profile. This includes a reduced seizure threshold and delirium, which may make it less useful in the elderly. Pethidine should be avoided.

Non-steroidal anti-inflammatory drugs (NSAIDs) pose particular problems in the elderly. There is a greater risk of gastrointestinal, cardiovascular and renal adverse effects. These drugs should be avoided where possible, and if used, only for the shortest possible time with the lowest possible dose and close monitoring.

Digoxin

Digoxin has a narrow therapeutic index and its pharmacokinetics are altered in the elderly (decreased volume of distribution, reduced clearance), making toxicity a potential problem. Both loading and maintenance doses should be reduced, with a maximum maintenance dose of 125 micrograms suggested (half of the normal maximum dose).

Anticoagulants

Elderly patients are more sensitive to the effects of warfarin, and at greater risk from adverse effects. However, it is also often omitted unnecessarily in elderly patients with atrial fibrillation who may benefit from it. Use of decision making tools (e.g. the CHADS$_2$ score) may help in careful consideration of the benefit/risk ratio for individual patients. Particular risks may be: possible interactions with antiplatelet drugs, risk factors for gastrointestinal bleeding and tendency to falls. If warfarin is used, lower loading doses are recommended, and it is likely lower maintenance doses will be required.

Antihypertensive drugs

Elderly patients will have lower resting heart rate and decreased tachycardic response to postural changes. They are therefore more susceptible to the bradycardic and hypotensive effects of many drugs. Angiotensin-converting enzyme inhibitors are less useful in the elderly and may cause increased renal impairment. Calcium channel blockers may contribute to constipation. Both verapamil and diltiazem have increased antihypertensive effects.

Anticholinergic drugs

Many different drug classes have anticholinergic effects (e.g. antihistamines, antidepressants and neuroleptics) that can be more pronounced in the elderly. Urinary retention, constipation and postural hypotension can be problematic. Try to avoid multiple anticholinergics in combination.

Antibiotics

Antibiotic associated diarrhoea and *Clostridium difficile* infection are more common in the elderly. Adverse effects of antibiotics such as delirium, seizures, haematological abnormalities and renal damage are also more common than in younger patients.

18 Prescribing in pregnancy and breast feeding

Figure 18.1 Stage of pregnancy and type of harm.
Note: Blue bars indicate time periods when major morphological abnormalities can occur, whereas light blue bars correspond to periods at risk for minor abnormalities and function defects.
CNS, central nervous system

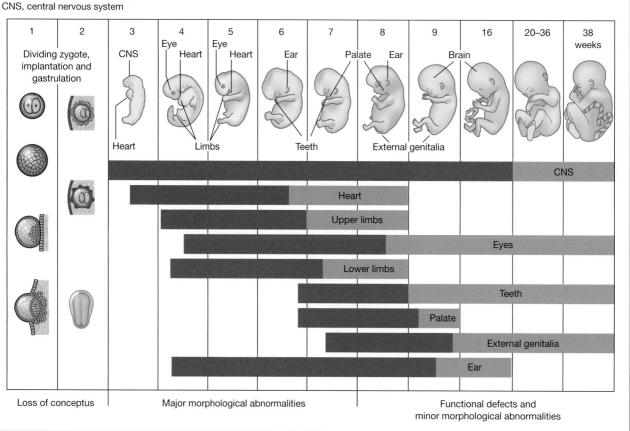

Prescribing at a Glance, First Edition. Sarah Ross. © 2014 John Wiley & Sons, Ltd. Published 2014 by John Wiley & Sons, Ltd.

Companion website: www.ataglanceseries.com/prescribing

What is different in pregnancy/ breast feeding

Pharmacokinetic and pharmacodynamic processes are altered by pregnancy, but perhaps more importantly, the effect of any drug on the fetus must be taken into consideration. In mothers who are breast feeding, consideration of whether the child will be exposed to the drug, and what consequences this may have, is important. Unfortunately, data on these aspects may not be available because of the lack of clinical trials in pregnant or breast feeding patients. Most data comes from observational studies, and so there may be more information about older drugs.

Pharmacokinetic changes in pregnancy

Changes to pharmacokinetics vary by trimester and are complex. In general, the following effects are seen, but adjustments must take the stage of pregnancy and other individual variation into account.

Gastric emptying may be delayed as pregnancy continues, which may increase the time to maximum concentration of a drug. Gastric pH increases and may affect bioavailability of some medicines. Perhaps more importantly, the nausea and vomiting of early pregnancy may make use of the oral route more challenging.

Volume of distribution is increased for a range of drugs because of the increase in total body water and fat stores as well as the reduction in plasma proteins. This can result in prolonged drug action.

The effects of pregnancy on metabolism vary between drugs. Some liver enzyme activity is increased, whereas other activity is reduced. In these instances, increases or decreases in dose may be needed.

Glomerular filtration rate increases by approximately 50%. This can increase the clearance of many renally excreted drugs. Dose adjustments may be needed.

Pharmacodynamic changes in pregnancy

Although it is recognised that changes occur, these are not well understood. Blood flow to tissues is altered, as is receptor function. The clinical implications are not clear.

Effects on the fetus

Again available data may be limited. Most drugs will cross the placenta, exposing the fetus to a range of possible effects (Figure 18.1). In the first trimester, teratogenicity may lead to congenital malformations as fetal organs develop. In the second and third trimesters, growth may be affected and some drugs may be fetotoxic. This can lead to carcinogenesis, organ damage and even death.

Breast feeding

Many substances ingested by lactating women are present in breast milk, although the levels tend to be less than *in utero*. It is important to know both the likely concentration and the potential effects in order to estimate risk.

Selecting medicines and regimes in pregnancy and breast feeding

Where possible, try to use non-pharmacological treatments. If a drug is needed, choose the option with the best safety record (this may be an older drug as data may be lacking for new drugs). Check on the most up-to-date information from the manufacturer by consulting the Schedule of Product Characteristics. Other information is available including data from the UK Teratology Information Service (UKTIS).

Use the lowest effective dose for the shortest possible time. Avoid the first 10 weeks of pregnancy if possible and consider stopping or reducing dose before delivery as there may be risks to both mother and fetus (e.g. increased bleeding from anticoagulants).

In general, drugs that are safe in children under 2 years of age are safe in breast feeding, but if possible choose drugs that are present in breast milk at lower concentrations. Information is available from LactMed produced by the US National Library of Medicine.

It is critical not to under treat maternal disease, which may pose a higher risk to mother and fetus than the risks of drug use. It is wise to optimise treatment of chronic conditions prior to pregnancy where possible to ensure good disease control and use of the safest possible therapy.

Remember to consider the effects of a therapy in pregnancy when prescribing for women of childbearing age, as many pregnancies are unplanned.

Specific medicines

Commonly used drugs which prescribers should be aware of are:

• Anticoagulants: warfarin is teratogenic and fetotoxic and should be avoided. Low molecular weight heparin is safe and can be used instead. Newer agents have not demonstrated safety.

• Antiplatelets: aspirin is safe in pregnancy, but may increase the risk of bleeding at delivery and should be avoided in breast feeding because of the risk of Reye's syndrome. There is no data for clopidogrel.

• Antihypertensives: methyldopa is the agent of choice as it has a long track record of safety; other agents may be used although there are some concerns. Angiotensin-converting enzyme (ACE) inhibitors and angiotensin II antagonists are contraindicated because of fetotoxicity.

• Anticonvulsants: congenital malformations are associated with many older anticonvulsants and safety is not established in newer agents. Treatment of epilepsy in pregnancy is important and should be undertaken by a specialist.

• Antidiabetic agents: current guidance suggests that any woman with pre-existing diabetes be switched to insulin and monitored by a specialist during pregnancy.

• Antibiotics: some classes are thought to be safe, such as penicillins and cephalosporins, others are known to be harmful, including tetracyclines and quinolones. Information should be sought about individual illnesses and agents.

• Analgesics: paracetamol is thought to be safe in pregnancy and breast feeding. Non-steroidal anti-inflammatory drugs (NSAIDs) should be avoided in pregnancy, but ibuprofen is thought to be safe in breast feeding. Opiates are harmful, but may be used with care in some circumstances.

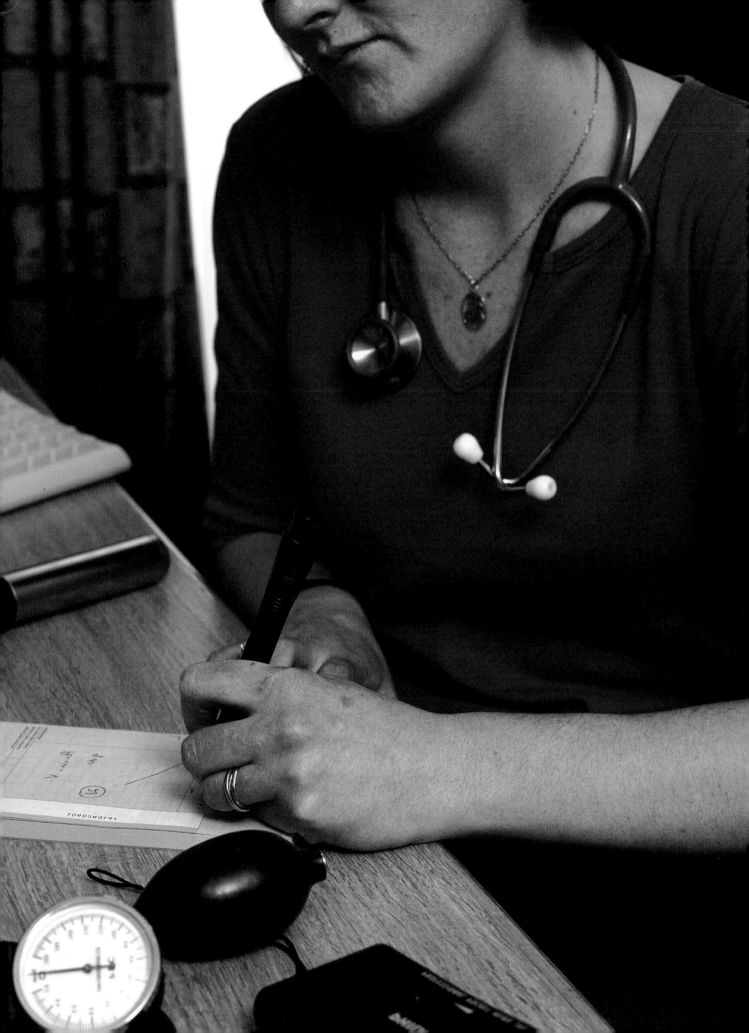

Logistics of prescribing

Part 4

Chapters

Don't forget to visit the companion website for this book www.ataglanceseries.com/prescribing to do some practice MCQs and case studies on these topics.

19 How to write a drug prescription

Figure 19.1   Hospital A.

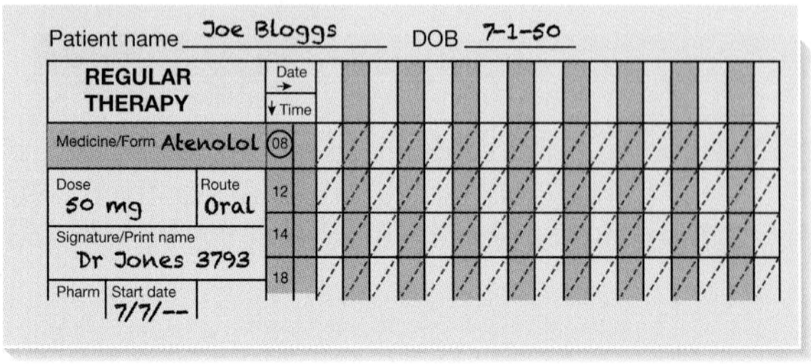

| Patient name | Joe Bloggs | DOB | 7-1-50 |

REGULAR THERAPY — Date / Time

Medicine/Form **Atenolol** (08)

Dose **50 mg**   Route **Oral**

Signature/Print name **Dr Jones 3793**

Pharm   Start date **7/7/--**

Figure 19.2   Hospital B.

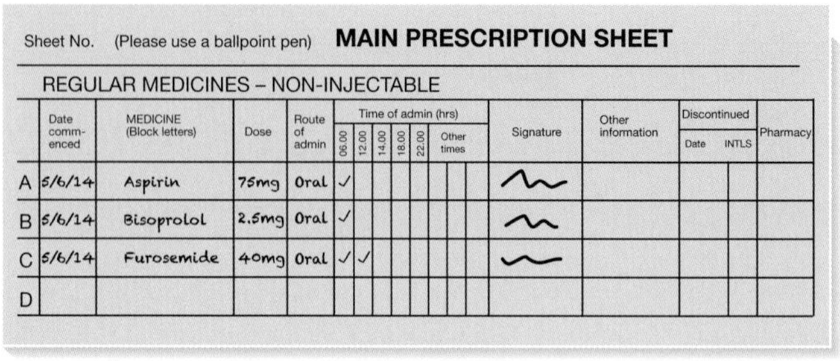

Sheet No.   (Please use a ballpoint pen)   **MAIN PRESCRIPTION SHEET**

REGULAR MEDICINES – NON-INJECTABLE

	Date commenced	MEDICINE (Block letters)	Dose	Route of admin	Time of admin (hrs) 06.00	12.00	14.00	18.00	22.00	Other times	Signature	Other information	Discontinued Date	INTLS	Pharmacy
A	5/6/14	Aspirin	75mg	Oral	✓						～				
B	5/6/14	Bisoprolol	2.5mg	Oral	✓						～				
C	5/6/14	Furosemide	40mg	Oral	✓	✓					～				
D															

Figure 19.3   Controlled drug prescription.

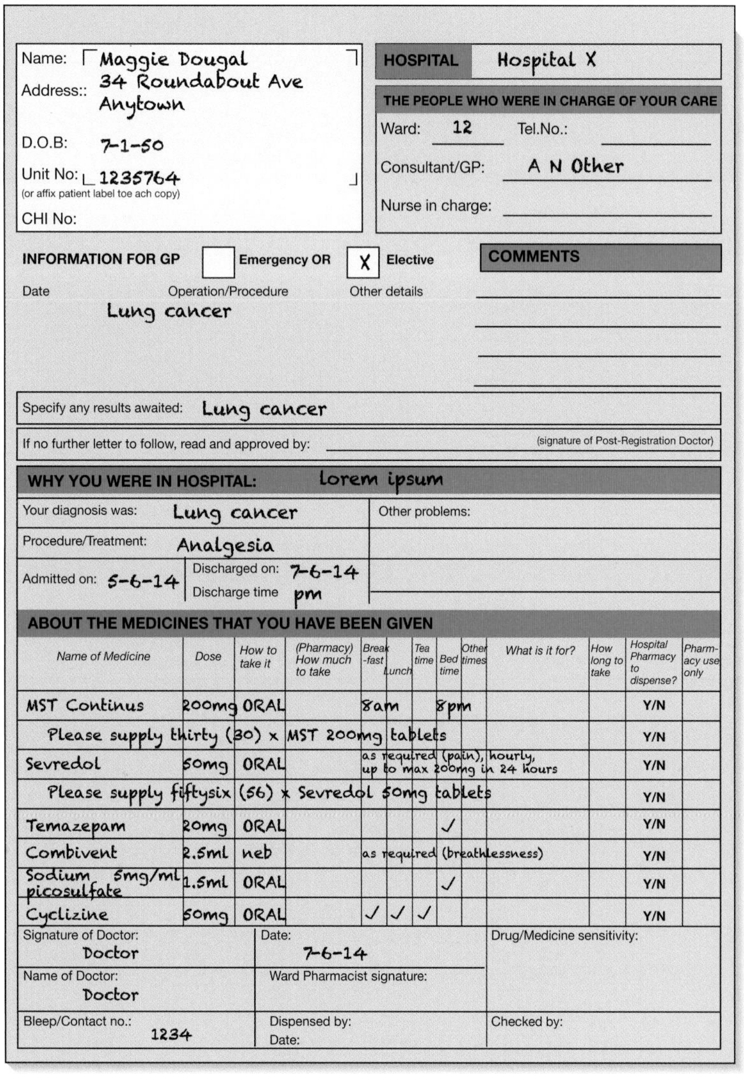

Name: Maggie Dougal
Address:: 34 Roundabout Ave
Anytown
D.O.B: 7-1-50
Unit No: 1235764
(or affix patient label to each copy)
CHI No:

HOSPITAL   Hospital X

THE PEOPLE WHO WERE IN CHARGE OF YOUR CARE
Ward: 12   Tel.No.:
Consultant/GP: A N Other
Nurse in charge:

INFORMATION FOR GP   [ ] Emergency OR   [X] Elective   COMMENTS

Date   Operation/Procedure   Other details
Lung cancer

Specify any results awaited: Lung cancer

If no further letter to follow, read and approved by: _____   (signature of Post-Registration Doctor)

WHY YOU WERE IN HOSPITAL: lorem ipsum

Your diagnosis was: Lung cancer   Other problems:

Procedure/Treatment: Analgesia

Admitted on: 5-6-14   Discharged on: 7-6-14   Discharge time pm

ABOUT THE MEDICINES THAT YOU HAVE BEEN GIVEN

Name of Medicine	Dose	How to take it	(Pharmacy) How much to take	Break-fast	Lunch	Tea time	Bed time	Other times	What is it for?	How long to take	Hospital Pharmacy to dispense?	Pharmacy use only
MST Continus	200mg	ORAL		8am			8pm				Y/N	
Please supply thirty (30) x MST 200mg tablets											Y/N	
Sevredol	50mg	ORAL			as required (pain), hourly, up to max 200mg in 24 hours						Y/N	
Please supply fiftysix (56) x Sevredol 50mg tablets											Y/N	
Temazepam	20mg	ORAL					✓				Y/N	
Combivent	2.5ml	neb			as required (breathlessness)						Y/N	
Sodium picosulfate 5mg/ml	1.5ml	ORAL					✓				Y/N	
Cyclizine	50mg	ORAL		✓	✓	✓					Y/N	

Signature of Doctor: Doctor   Date: 7-6-14   Drug/Medicine sensitivity:

Name of Doctor: Doctor   Ward Pharmacist signature:

Bleep/Contact no.: 1234   Dispensed by: Date: Checked by:

Figure 19.4   FP10 form.

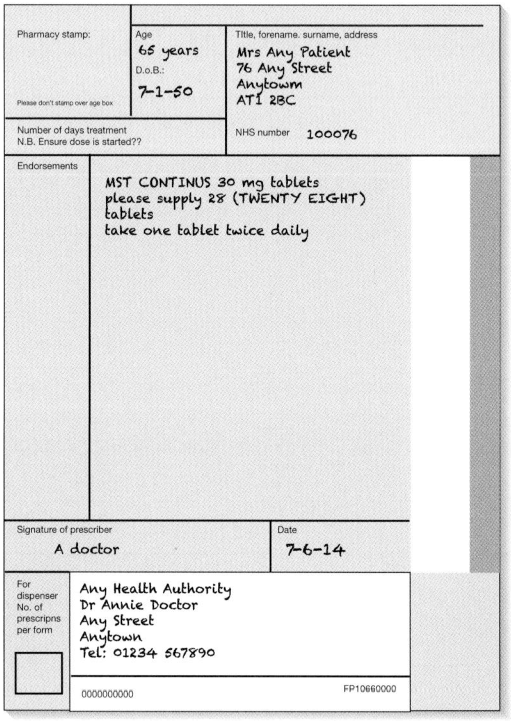

Pharmacy stamp:

Age 65 years   D.o.B.: 7-1-50   Please don't stamp over age box

Title, forename. surname, address
Mrs Any Patient
76 Any Street
Anytown
AT1 2BC

Number of days treatment N.B. Ensure dose is started??   NHS number   100076

Endorsements
MST CONTINUS 30 mg tablets
please supply 28 (TWENTY EIGHT) tablets
take one tablet twice daily

Signature of prescriber   A doctor   Date   7-6-14

For dispenser No. of prescripns per form

Any Health Authority
Dr Annie Doctor
Any Street
Anytown
Tel: 01234 567890

0000000000   FP10660000

General rules

It is critical that prescriptions are written correctly. This is important for patient safety and the correct supply of medicines, but also to prevent fraud.

All prescriptions should include sufficient details to accurately identify the patient, preferably name, address and date of birth (plus age for children under 12 years of age).

A prescription should include:
- Drug name
- Dose
- Route
- Frequency
- Any special instructions on how to take
- Prescriber's signature and date.

You must sign the prescription in ink (computerised prescriptions are increasingly used, and electronic signature may be permitted in some of these).

Other general rules are set out in the *British National Formulary* (BNF), including:
- Do not use decimal points unless needed (i.e. 1 mg rather than 1.0 mg); but the leading 0 must be used (i.e. 0.5 mL)
- Use grams where dose is more than 1 g, but milligrams where it is less (i.e. 500 mg, not 0.5 g); similarly use milligrams if more than 1 mg rather than micrograms
- Micrograms and nanograms should be written in full rather than as abbreviations
- Units should be written in full
- If 'as required' medicines are given, minimum dose frequency should be stated along with a maximum daily dose where relevant.

Some hospitals will have lists of acceptable abbreviations which should be used.

Prescriptions in secondary care
Inpatient charts

At present, most hospitals have their own unique prescription charts (often called kardexes). It is really important to be aware of this, and to ensure that these are correctly used when moving between different hospitals. Two main types are seen. In Figure 19.1, the administration record is on the same chart, in Figure 19.2 a separate chart is used. It is worthwhile becoming familiar with how administration is documented in order to know whether the medicine has been given. Many systems use numbers to indicate that a drug has not been administered and why. Kardex systems may include supplementary charts for anticoagulants, diabetic medicines, dermatological preparations, etc. It is important that everyone caring for the patient is aware of supplementary charts, so it may be good practice to write all drug names on the main chart and refer to the supplementary one.

It can be difficult to identify staff from a signature on a prescription and it is good practice to print your name alongside (and add bleep number if possible).

Discharge prescriptions

Errors can easily occur at the interface between primary and secondary care. The discharge prescription often has two purposes. Firstly, to instruct the pharmacist to dispense any medicines that the patient needs to take home. Secondly, the prescription provides the GP (and sometimes the patient) with a record of current medicines. Both these purposes should be borne in mind. A complete prescription that meets legal requirements is required for a pharmacist to dispense medicines. Some additional information may be needed by the GP to continue safely prescribing for the patient. This may be an instruction to titrate a dose, the intended duration of treatment or other information. If medicines have been stopped in hospital it is worth commenting on this to avoid any potential confusion by the patient or GP about whether this was intentional or in error. For specific medicines, supplementary information may be needed (e.g. warfarin). The prescriber who is continuing to prescribe this drug needs to know current and recent doses, as well as recent international normalised ratio (INR) results in order to prescribe safely and effectively.

Controlled drug prescriptions

Controlled drugs include many opiates and benzodiazepines. They are indicated in the BNF by this symbol (**CD**). These are drugs where the supply, possession, prescribing and record keeping are regulated by law (Misuse of Drugs Regulations 2001). All prescribers should be aware of these regulations. In hospital settings, controlled drugs can be prescribed in the same manner as other medicines; however, the storage and administration are closely monitored. Hospital practitioners need to follow controlled drug prescription rules for discharge prescriptions. These rules are also in place for primary care prescriptions. Pharmacists cannot legally dispense medicines unless all the requirements are met.

The prescription must:
- Be indelible
- Be signed by the prescriber
- Be dated
- Specify the prescriber's address
- Specify name and address of the patient
- State the form and strength of the preparation
- State the total quantity (in both words and figures).

An example is shown in Figure 19.3.

Prescriptions in primary care

Primary care prescriptions are written (or printed by an electronic system) on statutory forms (FP10 in England [Figure 19.4], GP10 in Scotland, WP10 in Wales and HS21 in Northern Ireland). These should be written as shown. Any extra space should be cancelled out to avoid fraudulent addition of medicines.

20 Communicating with patients about medicines

Figure 20.1 Example of a visual aid. TPA, Tissue plasminogen activator.
(Adapted from Medscape)

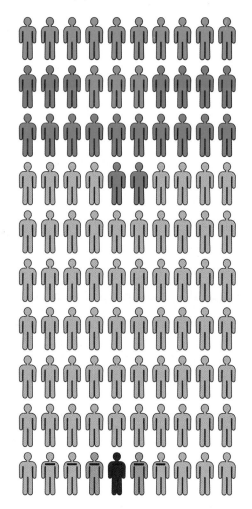

TPA for cerebral ischaemia within 3 hours of onset: changes in outcome due to treatment

- Normal or nearly normal
- Better
- No major change
- Worse
- Severely disabled or dead

Early course:
- No early worsening with brain bleeding
- Early worsening with brain bleeding

Giving information

Patients need information about new medicines, including the name and nature of the medicine and the reasons for taking it, side effects to be aware of and when the treatment will be reviewed. In addition, patients should be given an idea of how long the medicine will take to start working, what the medicine should do and how they can tell whether it is effective or not. They also need practical information on how and when to take the medication and about any common interactions (e.g. alcohol) or activities to avoid (e.g. driving). Making decisions about the amount of information to give, particularly about side effects, is challenging. It is not practical to give all possible information and patients will vary in the amount of information that they want. You should try to tailor explanations to the patient's needs. Studies have suggested that patients often want more information about possible side effects than doctors give, so it may help to specifically ask a patient what they want to know. This can be a good opportunity to encourage patients to be more engaged with their treatment.

Information should be given in appropriate sized chunks, following which you should check the patient's level of understanding. Some degree of repetition may be needed to ensure important information is retained. Care must be taken not to overload the patient with verbal information that they might not remember. Written information in the form of patient information leaflets or other documentation may allow prescribers to mention only the most important information while still ensuring the patient can access full information. Alternatively, it may be helpful to write down the critical information for the patient.

It is usually wise to describe common side effects and what to do about them (if anything). It is also important to warn patients about any serious effects (although these are often rare) and circumstances in which they should contact a doctor. This information can be found in the *British National Formulary* (where side effects are listed in order of frequency) and the Schedule of Product Characteristics (which often lists side effects by body system and then gives an indication of how common they are). You will generally become more confident about which side effects to discuss as you become more familiar with the medicine in question. Patients may overestimate the risk of side effects if these are described in qualitative terms. Giving numerical estimates to quantify 'common' or 'uncommon' effects may improve understanding.

Be aware that patients may use a range of sources to obtain information about medicines, and you may wish to direct patients to reputable sources.

Shared decision making

Shared decision making or concordance describes a process where patients are partners in decisions about medicines (Box 20.1). This process has been shown to increase patient satisfaction with the consultation and is considered useful for maximising adherence. Not all patients or treatment decisions are appropriate for this process, however. Some patients may not wish to be involved in decisions, preferring a more traditional model of consultation, or they may not be able to participate because of cultural, educational or cognitive factors. It is important that you can identify when a decision should be shared, and you should have the skills to guide the patient.

In order to facilitate shared decision making, prescribers need to be able to convey information about risks and benefits of treatment. This can be challenging to do in an objective and unbiased way, as well as to source appropriate information in the first place. Remember that doctors' own estimations of risk and benefit are prone to bias and be aware that the way in which risk is discussed can influence the patient's beliefs. There are some simple ways in which the presentation of risk can be improved:

• Avoid descriptive terms alone: terms such as 'uncommon' can be interpreted in a variety of ways.

• Give the probability of possible outcomes with the same denominator, for example, 1 in 100 and 5 in 100. If different denominators are used, patients may be confused.

• Offer both positive and negative outcomes: this will avoid the 'framing effect' (where presenting the negative outcome can carry more weight in the same situation than giving the positive outcome, for example, 'one in five patients experience a side effect' versus 'four out of five patients have no side effects').

• Use absolute numbers: the relative risk will often have larger numbers and can be more persuasive than the absolute risk (e.g. a 25% relative risk reduction may equate to an absolute risk reduction of 1% from 4% to 3%).

• Use visual aids where available (for an example, see Figure 20.1). Sources of information about risks and benefits can be found in guidelines such as those produced by the National Institute for Health and Care Excellence (NICE), publications such as *Clinical Evidence* by the *British Medical Journal* and information produced by speciality bodies. Be wary of sources of information that may be biased (e.g. promotional pharmaceutical information) or presented in such a way as to emphasise benefits.

(21) Therapeutic drug monitoring

Figure 21.1   Steady-state concentration.

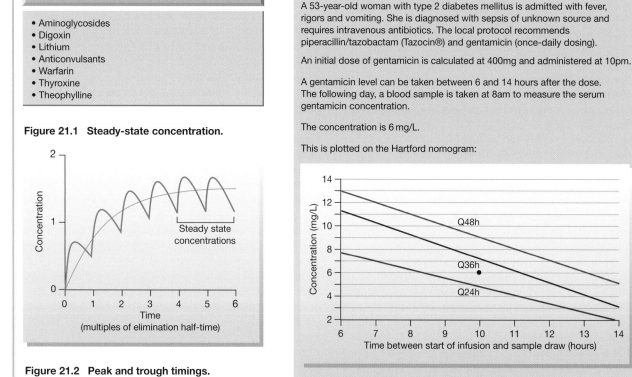

Figure 21.2   Peak and trough timings.

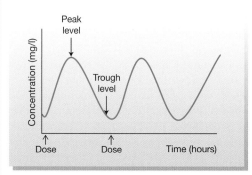

Box 21.2   Gentamicin monitoring

A 53-year-old woman with type 2 diabetes mellitus is admitted with fever, rigors and vomiting. She is diagnosed with sepsis of unknown source and requires intravenous antibiotics. The local protocol recommends piperacillin/tazobactam (Tazocin®) and gentamicin (once-daily dosing).

An initial dose of gentamicin is calculated at 400 mg and administered at 10pm.

A gentamicin level can be taken between 6 and 14 hours after the dose. The following day, a blood sample is taken at 8am to measure the serum gentamicin concentration.

The concentration is 6 mg/L.

This is plotted on the Hartford nomogram:

The level is plotted within the 36-hour dosing area, so the next dose of gentamicin (same dose) is prescribed for 10am the following day. A further level should be taken within 6 to 14 hours of this dose and the same process followed.

Prescribing at a Glance, First Edition. Sarah Ross. © 2014 John Wiley & Sons, Ltd. Published 2014 by John Wiley & Sons, Ltd.
Companion website: www.ataglanceseries.com/prescribing

Common medicines where therapeutic drug monitoring is used

Therapeutic drug monitoring (TDM) is the process of measuring drug concentration. It is commonly used when there is significant inter-patient variation in drug concentration (caused by differences in absorption, metabolism and elimination) to allow prescribers to individualise drug doses. This is most important where drugs have a narrow therapeutic index (i.e. a small difference between the therapeutic and toxic concentrations). In addition, it is most useful when there is difficulty in interpreting the difference between therapeutic and toxic effects clinically, a clear relationship between drug concentration and effect, and a lack of active metabolites. In practice, TDM is only routinely used for a small range of drugs (Box 21.1).

While TDM is primarily used to individualise therapy or detect toxicity, it can also be used to ensure that a therapeutic concentration is reached or to assess patient compliance.

Practicalities of measuring plasma drug concentrations

The timing of sampling is critical in ensuring that a usable measurement is taken. Firstly, enough time must have passed for a steady state to be established (Figure 21.1). This is normally considered to be after five half-lives (e.g. digoxin is thought to have a half-life of about 30 to 40 hours, and so a steady-state level will be reached after at least 5×30 to 40 hours or 6 to 8 days). Secondly, care must be taken about how long after a dose the level is taken. Three types of level are taken, depending on the drug: a peak level, a trough level or a level during the dose interval (Figure 21.2). A peak level is taken after the dose is administered. A trough level is normally taken just prior to the next dose. These levels are commonly used in antibiotic monitoring. Other levels can be taken during the dose interval, depending on the half-life of the drug. There is generally guidance available on the timing (e.g. digoxin can be measured 6 hours after administration). It is vital that the time of sampling is recorded. This allows for correct interpretation. In modern healthcare, it is highly likely that the practitioner taking the blood sample and the one interpreting it are different. This makes documentation all the more important.

How to interpret drug concentration

The initial step in interpreting a drug concentration is to ensure that the sample is appropriate for the question being asked. For example, if toxicity is suspected, a level outside the accepted trough range may indicate this. If poor compliance is suspected, a low or undetectable level after dosing may provide evidence to support these concerns.

Remember that other information may be needed to interpret a drug concentration. This may include patient age, gender, renal function or other factors. All interpretation should be made with the individual patient's clinical state in mind.

The laboratory used should provide a reference range for the drug, but these are also available in the product literature and in journal articles. Local guidance may be available, particularly for antibiotic prescribing.

If the sample has been taken at an appropriate time, it is straightforward to tell whether the drug concentration is within the recommended range. This information should then be considered in the light of the patient's overall condition. If necessary, a dose adjustment can be made.

How to adjust dosage

If the drug concentration is not appropriate, there are two ways of changing it. Most often, the dose is adjusted; however, it is also possible to manipulate the drug concentration by changing the dosing frequency (see Chapters 7 and 8).

In the case of toxicity, it may be necessary to stop the drug, and then to consider whether it should be restarted, when and at what dose.

It is possible in some cases to calculate what the new dose should be in order to achieve the desired concentration. It may be helpful to ask for help from a pharmacist or senior colleague. In some instances, guidance on dose changes may be available from local guidance or drug information sources.

Once a dose change has occurred, plans should be put in place to recheck the drug level as appropriate. For some drugs, regular TDM will be required (i.e. warfarin), whereas for others once a suitable dose is found (i.e. digoxin), no further checks are needed unless the situation changes.

22 Dealing with adverse drug reactions

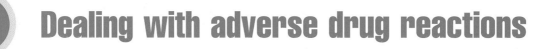

Figure 22.1 Yellow Card reporting form. (Source: Reproduced with permission from the Medicines and Healthcare Products Regulatory Agency.)

Box 22.1 Identifying an adverse drug reaction

Timing: does the time course of the reaction fit with when the medicine was started (and stopped)?
Plausibility: does the reaction fit with the known pharmacology of the drug (is it a type A reaction)?
Corroborating data: has this adverse effect been reported before?
Re-challenge: does the adverse drug reaction stop when the medicine is discontinued, and does it recur on re-challenge with the medicine?

Prescribing at a Glance, First Edition. Sarah Ross. © 2014 John Wiley & Sons, Ltd. Published 2014 by John Wiley & Sons, Ltd.
Companion website: www.ataglanceseries.com/prescribing

Adverse drug reactions

An adverse drug reaction (ADR) is 'any undesirable effect of a drug beyond its anticipated therapeutic effects occurring during clinical use'. ADRs are common, causing approximately 5% of admissions to hospital and occurring in 10% to 20% of all hospital inpatients. They lead to substantial morbidity and mortality.

ADRs are subcategorised in a variety of ways, but the most helpful distinction is between type A (predictable) and type B (unpredictable). Type A reactions are dose related and are caused by the known pharmacological properties of the drug, whereas type B are not dose related and thought to be caused by immunological reactions. This means that many ADRs can be predicted and should be obvious to spot in patients. Many ADRs are caused by a small group of commonly used drugs such as antibiotics, anticoagulants, diuretics and non-steroidal anti-inflammatory drugs. You should be alert to common ADRs when using these medicines. In addition, certain patients are at greater risk of experiencing an ADR. Risk factors include age, female gender and multiple drug regimens.

How to identify an adverse drug reaction

Prescribers should consider an ADR as a differential diagnosis in any patient who presents with new symptoms. An ADR is easy to identify when it is a commonly recognised problem with a drug that the patient is taking. However, many cases are not so clear cut. Prescribers can rarely be 100% certain that a particular medicine has caused a particular reaction. Considering a number of factors can help (Box 22.1):

- Timing: does the time course of the reaction fit with when the medicine was started (and stopped)? A symptom that precedes the drug is unlikely to be related, but one that occurs soon after could be. Remember that some ADRs can present long after the initiation of a drug (e.g. corticosteroids causing osteoporosis).
- Plausibility: does the reaction fit with the known pharmacology of the drug (is it a type A reaction)? If it does, the link is easier to make.
- Corroborating data: has this adverse effect been reported before (check sources of information like the *British National Formulary* and the Schedule of Product Characteristics)?
- Re-challenge: does the ADR stop when the medicine is discontinued, and recur on re-challenge with the medicine? However, it may be that the ADR is so severe that re-challenge is not wise.

Managing an adverse drug reaction

If an ADR is suspected, you must choose whether to continue with the drug, reduce the dose or stop it. Some ADRs are transient and will disappear if the patient persists with the drug for a few days (e.g. nausea with antibiotics). Other ADRs are likely to persist throughout the course of treatment (e.g. constipation with opiates).

A number of considerations are important when deciding how to manage the patient: the severity of the ADR, the severity of the disease being treated, the availability of alternative drugs and the patient's preference. Some mild side effects may be tolerable, particularly if the medicine is effective and there are few other good options. At the other extreme, some ADRs are highly dangerous and the drug should be stopped and not used again (e.g. anaphylaxis). If the ADRs is a type A reaction, reducing the dose of the drug may reduce the unwanted effect. Type B reactions will not respond in this way.

Some ADRs can be managed using other drugs. For example, constipation with opiates is common and can be managed with laxatives. Where possible, however, it is wise to keep the number of drugs to a minimum and avoid a 'prescribing cascade' where drugs are added to others to treat side effects.

Reporting an adverse drug reaction

Reporting ADRs is a critical part of ensuring drug safety and is the duty of all prescribers. Many adverse effects are only seen when drugs are used in large numbers of patients, rather than in clinical trials that may have only included a few thousand patients, so it is vital to have systems to monitor new drugs after licensing. Reporting systems attempt to identify new ADRs and to clarify the incidence/severity of ADRs. Reporting in the UK is performed through the 'yellow card' system. Firstly, any suspected ADR in a new drug (as demarcated by the black triangle in the *British National Formulary* [BNF]), should be reported whether noted before and regardless of the severity. Secondly, any serious reaction with an established drug should be reported (e.g. if it is fatal, life threatening, causes or prolongs hospital admission). It is not necessary for you to be completely certain about whether the symptom is an ADR, as this is assessed by experts who have access to any similar reports and can therefore triangulate several sources of data.

Yellow Card forms (Figure 22.1) are found in the paper copies of the BNF and BNF for Children and are also available online at https://yellowcard.mhra.gov.uk/. The scheme is open to other healthcare professionals and now to patients. When reporting a possible ADR, the following information is needed: brief patient details, the name of the suspected drug plus all other medicines taken concurrently by the patient, and a description of the suspected reaction including its outcome.

23 Avoiding drug interactions (drugs, food and alternative medicines)

Table 23.1 Interactions with cytochrome P450

CYP1A2	CYP2C9	CYP2C19	CYP2D6	CYP3A4
Inducers				
Smoking	Rifampicin		St John's Wort	Carbamazepine
			Phenytoin	
			Rifampicin	
Inhibitors				
Ciprofloxacin	Amiodarone	Fluoxetine	Duloxetine	Indinavir
Ofloxacin	Fluconazole	Omeprazole	Fluoxetine	Ritonavir
Levofloxacin	Isoniazide	Lansoprazole	Paroxetine	Clarithromycin
Amiodarone		Ketoconazole	Amiodarone	Erythromycin
		Chlorphenamine	Fluconazole	
		Clomipramine	Itraconazole	
		Ritonavir	Ketoconazole	
			Diltiazem	
			Verapamil	

Box 23.1 Drugs commonly targets for interactions

- Warfarin
- Theophylline
- Gentamicin
- Digoxin
- Lithium
- Phenytoin

Box 23.1 Drugs commonly involved in interactions

- Antibacterials, particularly macrolides, quinolones, antifungals
- Anticonvulsants, particularly phenytoin, carbamazepine, valproate
- Drugs that reduce glomerular filtration rate, particularly angiotensin-converting enzyme inhibitors/ angiotensin receptor blockers, diuretics, non-steroidal anti-inflammatory drugs

Prescribing at a Glance, First Edition. Sarah Ross. © 2014 John Wiley & Sons, Ltd. Published 2014 by John Wiley & Sons, Ltd.
Companion website: www.ataglanceseries.com/prescribing

Drug interactions

The effects of many drugs can be changed by substances such as other drugs, food, cigarettes and alternative medicines. Drug interactions can be pharmacokinetic or pharmacodynamic and are not always harmful or clinically important. It is important that you are aware of potential interactions; however, it is not sensible to try to remember all of them, rather you should know when to suspect them and which references to consult to check. In addition, it is helpful to be aware of interactions with common drugs such as warfarin where serious problems can arise.

Interaction mechanisms

Interactions can occur at any stage in the pharmacokinetic processes of administration, distribution, metabolism and excretion. Many of the most important interactions are at the metabolism or excretion stages. The end result is a change in the drug concentration, which will give either a reduced or increased (possibly toxic) effect. Clearly, interactions with drugs that have narrow therapeutic indices (a small difference between the effective and toxic concentrations) are more likely to be problematic.

Pharmacodynamic interactions occur when a drug's effect is changed by the presence of another substance at the site of action. These can be antagonistic or synergistic effects on either the desired effect or adverse effects of the drug. They should be considered when drugs have similar effects.

Predicting interactions

Important pharmacokinetic interactions are generally seen in drugs with narrow therapeutic indices. The most common are listed in Box 23.1. These interactions are either caused by substances that induce or inhibit the metabolism of drugs by the hepatic cytochrome P450 enzyme system (common culprits include various antimicrobial and anticonvulsant agents; see Table 23.1) or because of interference with renal excretion (Box 23.2). Any substance that reduces the glomerular filtration rate may cause toxicity from renally excreted drugs. Commonly used drugs that are potentially nephrotoxic include non-steroidal anti-inflammatory drugs, angiotensin-converting enzyme inhibitors and diuretics.

Pharmacodynamic interactions are more difficult to predict, but should be considered when drugs with the potential to cause serious harm are used. For example, anticoagulant and antiplatelet drugs will interact with each other to increase the risk of bleeding. The other situation to be wary of is where drugs act antagonistically, for example beta receptor blockers and beta agonists.

Avoiding interactions

It is important to remember that drug interactions are not always with other drugs. Alcohol and smoking can cause pharmacokinetic interactions through the P450 enzyme system (Table 23.1). Various food stuffs, particularly cranberry juice and grapefruit have an effect on certain P450 enzymes. A range of alternative medicines such as St John's wort have been shown to interact at a pharmacokinetic level, and these are all the more dangerous as comprehensive data on interactions may not be available.

When prescribing a drug that can cause interactions (think of antimicrobials particularly) or be the target of these (listed above), you should look at the literature to identify potential interactions. The patient can then be more closely monitored to identify any problem that may arise or an alternative treatment can be chosen. Too often predictable interactions cause adverse reactions that could have been avoided.

Equally, when prescribing a less common drug that is unfamiliar to you, you should check for possible interactions.

Remember that it is possible to adjust the dose to allow for interactions when two substances are taken together over the long term (e.g. warfarin and amiodarone). Often problems are caused by short courses of therapy (e.g. antibiotics) or the occasional ingestion of alcohol/food stuffs rather than long-term co-prescribing.

Sources of information

The *British National Formulary* has an appendix on drug interactions (Appendix 1), which lists common interactions. The more critical ones are marked with a black dot to help identify them. The Schedule of Product Characteristics for each drug will also contain some information. Other texts listing interactions such as *Stockley's Drug Interactions* are more comprehensive (available to NHS staff online). Online websites are that list drugs metabolised by P450 liver enzymes are also available.

What to do if an interaction occurs

The first step in dealing with a drug interaction is to recognise it. In patients presenting with an adverse drug reaction, it is always worth considering whether this has been precipitated by an interaction. This may involve checking the literature. Suspicion should be aroused if a new medicine has been recently started.

Once identified, you must institute any required emergency treatment and then decide whether to stop one of the interacting drugs or to continue therapy at a lower dose. In doing so, the need for each treatment and its alternatives should be considered.

24 Avoiding prescribing errors

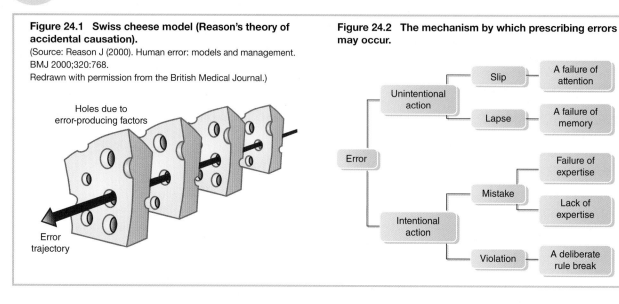

Figure 24.1 Swiss cheese model (Reason's theory of accidental causation).

(Source: Reason J (2000). Human error: models and management. BMJ 2000;320:768.

Redrawn with permission from the British Medical Journal.)

Holes due to error-producing factors

Error trajectory

Figure 24.2 The mechanism by which prescribing errors may occur.

Error

Unintentional action
- Slip — A failure of attention
- Lapse — A failure of memory

Intentional action
- Mistake — Failure of expertise
- Mistake — Lack of expertise
- Violation — A deliberate rule break

Why do errors happen?

There is now a great deal of research around error in healthcare. Prescribing errors are common (approximately 7% of prescribed items and 30% of patients in an inpatient setting). Most of these will not harm the patient, either because they are 'caught' and corrected or because the error itself does not cause harm. It is very difficult to predict which combinations of patient and drug factors lead to harm, and so it is wise to attempt to minimise error overall.

A key theory that can help explain why things go wrong, and guide interventions to reduce error, is Reason's theory of accidental causation (also known as human error theory or the 'Swiss cheese' model; see Figure 24.1). This model shows how factors in the systems in which we work can contribute to errors. To avoid making an error, 'holes' in the system should be plugged and extra defences can be added.

Errors can be unintentional (e.g. confusion over a drug name) or intentional (e.g. choosing the wrong drug) (Figure 24.2). Different types of error have different causes.

Error-producing factors exist in the work environment, the task, team, individuals and patients. Common issues include high workload, distractions and interruptions, poor communication, complex patients, high-risk drugs, lack of knowledge/experience and lack of adequate available information. Many of these are not within the control of individual prescribers, but being aware of high-risk situations can be helpful in avoiding error.

Extra defences are needed to reduce error. These can be checking procedures, whether by the prescriber themselves or by other staff. In studies, junior doctors often describe a lack of time or a sense of embarrassment that prevents them checking medicines information. In addition, they often assume that other staff members will check their prescriptions. Unfortunately this is not possible 7 days a week, 24 hours a day. It is critical that you act safely and check with sources such as the BNF or a pharmacist where needed.

Checking is also important when prescribing decisions are made by someone else and you are following instructions. These may not be as detailed as needed or they may even be wrong. It is sensible to ask for more information or clarification if required. Never write a prescription that you are unsure of.

Try to plan and prioritise work so that, where possible, prescribing is performed for one patient at a time without interruption and distraction. Concentrating on the task reduces the chance of error. Many prescriptions are left incomplete because the prescriber was distracted by another task. It is sensible to try to finish one task at a time; however, this can be very difficult in some working environments. It may even be worth regarding prescribing as a high-risk activity where you ask other team members not to interrupt you.

It is good practice to check for possible errors in any prescription when you are reviewing a chart or letter, whether this is in order to add a medicine or to transcribe a list of medicines. You can be a defence in the system by using these opportunities to look for and correct any errors.

Learning from error is vital in preventing future errors. It can be difficult to receive feedback on anything that goes wrong with a prescription you have written. It is well worth seeking out opportunities to learn from your own errors. Discussion of an error at a ward level can be useful, and gives you the chance to learn from each other. Patterns of error may reveal 'holes' in the system, and the team can consider how to address these issues. It is important to remember that identification and reporting of an error is not intended to attribute blame, but to provide data from which to learn.

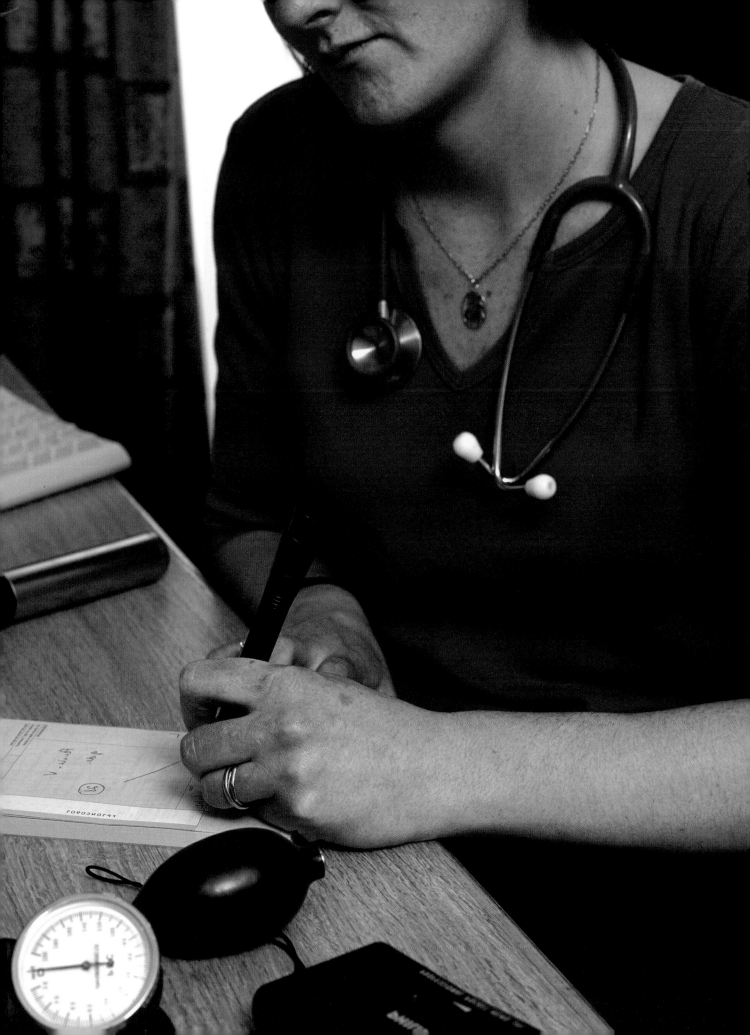

Specific drug groups

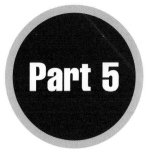

Part 5

Chapters

Don't forget to visit the companion website for this book
www.ataglanceseries.com/prescribing to do some
practice MCQs and case studies on these topics.

25 Using drugs for the gastrointestinal system

Table 25.1 Options for treating dyspepsia

Acid suppression	Efficacy	Problems
Antacids	Less effective	May reduce absorption of other medicines Diarrhoea/constipation
H$_2$-antagonists	Moderately effective	Diarrhoea
Proton pump inhibitors	Very effective	Diarrhoea Long-term use associated with *Clostridium difficile* infection and osteoporosis
Helicobacter eradication therapy	Effective if *Helicobacter* present	Side effects from antibiotics Compliance issues

Table 25.2 Suggested *Helicobacter pylori* eradication regimens[a]

Proton pump inhibitors (PPI)	PPI dose	Amoxicillin	Clarithromycin	Metronidazole
Lansoprazole	30 mg twice a day	1 g twice a day	500 mg twice a day	
	30 mg twice a day	1 g twice a day		400 mg twice a day
	30 mg twice a day		250 mg twice a day	400 mg twice a day
Omeprazole	20 mg twice a day	1 g twice a day	500 mg twice a day	
	20 mg twice a day	500 mg three times a day		400 mg three times a day
	20 mg twice a day		250 mg twice a day	400 mg twice a day
Pantoprazole	40 mg twice a day	1 g twice a day	500 mg twice a day	
	40 mg twice a day		250 mg twice a day	400 mg twice a day

[a]A 7 day course (14 days treatment will increase eradication rates, but poor compliance and adverse effects make this less useful)

Acid suppression

Dyspepsia is a common symptom. It may be a sign of serious disease so it is important that the correct diagnosis is made before starting acid suppression therapy. This means that prescribers should be alert to 'red flag' symptoms such as gastrointestinal bleeding, dysphagia, weight loss, abdominal swelling or persistent vomiting. Most dyspepsia is benign, however, caused by gastro-oesophageal reflux disease (GORD), uncomplicated peptic ulcer disease or non-ulcer dyspepsia.

The main groups of drugs are listed in Table 25.1. Non-pharmacological management and lifestyle change are important in reducing symptoms.

Antacids are widely used and very safe medicines containing magnesium or aluminium salts, which neutralise gastric acid and raise gastric pH, thereby increasing gastric emptying. They are less effective than other acid suppressants. In general, liquid preparations are more effective than tablets. Magnesium-containing antacids can cause diarrhoea, whereas those with aluminium may cause constipation. In patients with liver failure, the large sodium load may increase ascites and can precipitate constipation, leading to encephalopathy. Similarly, renal patients may experience fluid retention with aluminium salts or magnesium toxicity with magnesium salts. Antacids can affect the absorption of other drugs, so should not be taken at the same time of day.

H_2-Antagonists block histamine receptors that promote acid production by gastric parietal cells in response to gastrin. Ranitidine is the most commonly used agent, but the use of this class has been superseded by proton pump inhibitors (PPIs), which are more effective. H_2-Antagonists can cause diarrhoea, headache and dizziness infrequently, and occasionally cause a rash. The BNF lists a number of rare but important effects. Cimetidine can cause gynaecomastia and impotence, as well as interactions via the cytochrome P450 system, but is now very rarely used.

PPIs have revolutionised the treatment of GORD and peptic ulcer disease. They work by blocking the proton pump in the gastric parietal cell that moves hydrogen ions into the gut lumen where it forms hydrochloric acid. They are highly effective, but possibly overused. As with all treatments, the lowest effective dose should be used for the shortest possible duration. Higher doses are used for ulcer healing, but can be reduced after 4 to 8 weeks, depending on the indication. *Helicobacter pylori* eradication therapy may remove the need for further PPI prescription (Table 25.2).

Interactions with PPIs are partly group effects (i.e. interference with absorption of other drugs caused by raising stomach pH), but there are some drug-specific effects (i.e. interactions via cytochrome P450s). In general, omeprazole (and its enantiomer esomeprazole) has the most commonly seen issues, inhibiting a range of drugs including clopidogrel, warfarin and phenytoin.

Side effects include gastrointestinal upset and diarrhoea as well as headache. Importantly, use of PPIs is associated with an increased incidence of *Clostridium difficile* infection and osteoporotic fractures.

Antimotility drugs

These drugs work by increasing gut transit time through binding to opioid receptors in the gut. Antimotility drugs can be used in the management of chronic diarrhoea, particularly in irritable bowel disease. Treatment is not usually indicated in acute diarrhoea. Loperamide and codeine are the most commonly used drugs, although loperamide has the advantage of not crossing the blood–brain barrier and so avoiding central opioid side effects. Codeine should be avoided in renal impairment, and any antimotility drugs should be used with caution in diverticular disease. The main other adverse effect is abdominal cramping.

Laxatives

It is worth ensuring that the cause of constipation is addressed and that non-pharmacological measures (such as increased fluid and fibre intake) are instituted. It is also important to understand what the patient means by constipation. True constipation is the passing of hard stool less often than what is normal for the patient. Overuse of laxatives can be harmful, so they should be reserved for true constipation. Indications include irritable bowel syndrome, bowel preparation for procedures and avoidance of constipation associated with drugs. All laxatives (except softeners) should be avoided if bowel obstruction is suspected as this can lead to perforation.

Oral laxatives will take a few days to work. Rectal enemas will work more quickly. In hospital settings, it is sensible to ask experienced nurses for advice about bowel management. Common side effects of laxatives are nausea, abdominal discomfort and flatulence.

Bulk-forming laxatives (e.g. ispaghula hulk and sterculia) work by increasing the faecal mass in the same way as dietary fibre. They are generally prescribed once or twice a day, after meals. Rectal options are not available.

Faecal softeners work as softeners or lubricants. Glycerine suppositories are commonly used. Enemas, such as arachis oil are available. Arachis oil is derived from peanut oil so should be avoided in peanut allergy. Docusate has both softening and stimulating properties.

Stimulant laxatives (e.g. bisacodyl, senna) work by irritating the mucosa or sensory nerve endings. Prolonged use can damage these structures, and ideally the laxatives should only be used for short periods. Sodium picosulfate is very effective and usually reserved for bowel preparation. Dantron has been associated with carcinogenesis and should only be used for terminally ill patients. Cramping pain is more common with this type of laxative.

Osmotic laxatives (e.g. lactulose and macrogols) draw fluid into the gut lumen increasing stool bulk. For this reason they should be accompanied by adequate hydration. Cramping abdominal pain can be a problem.

Antispasmodics

Drugs that relax gut muscle can be useful in a variety of circumstances, but are mainly used for irritable bowel syndrome and in colicky abdominal pain. There are two groups of drugs: those that act on muscarinic receptors (dicycloverine, hyoscine) and those that are thought to have a direct relaxant effect on smooth muscle (mebeverine, peppermint oil). These are regarded as very safe and can be bought over the counter in pharmacies. The main adverse effects of antimuscarinics are well known and include constipation, urinary retention and dry mouth. They can cause confusion in the elderly. Allergic reactions are seen for all antispasmodics.

Remember that there are two types of hyoscine: butylbromide (Buscopan®) that is used in gastrointestinal disorders and hydrobromide that is a motion sickness treatment (Kwells®).

Using drugs for the cardiovascular system I

Table 26.1 Cardiovascular drug classes

Drug class	Mechanism of action	Indications	Major adverse effects
Loop diuretics (e.g. furosemide)	Inhibits NaCl reabsorption in the thick ascending loop of Henle	Heart failure	Electrolyte disturbance; dehydration/renal impairment
Thiazide diuretics (e.g. bendroflumethiazide)	Inhibits NaCl reabsorption in the distal tubule	Hypertension	Electrolyte disturbance; gout
Aldosterone antagonists (e.g. spironolactone)	Antagonises the effects of aldosterone	Heart failure; hypertension	Hyperkalaemia; gynaecomastia/breast enlargement
Beta blockers (e.g. atenolol)	Acts on beta-receptors in the sympathetic nervous system, reducing heart rate and cardiac output; mechanism in hypertension is unknown	Angina; heart failure; hypertension; tachyarrhythmias	Bradycardia; hypotension; cold peripheries; bronchospasm
Calcium channel blockers (e.g. amlodipine)	Blocks calcium channels causing relaxation of vascular smooth muscle relaxation	Angina; hypertension	Hypotension; flushing; headache; ankle swelling; bradycardia (verapamil and diltiazem)
Nitrates (e.g. GTN)	Causes release of nitric oxide, causing vascular smooth muscle	Angina; heart failure	Hypotension; flushing; headache

Prescribing at a Glance, First Edition. Sarah Ross. © 2014 John Wiley & Sons, Ltd. Published 2014 by John Wiley & Sons, Ltd.
Companion website: www.ataglanceseries.com/prescribing

Diuretics

Diuretics are very widely used drugs. They are divided into three main types: loop diuretics such as furosemide that are primarily used for heart failure and fluid overload, thiazide diuretics that are used for hypertension, and potassium-sparing diuretics that can be used for both.

Furosemide can be given orally or intravenously. If given intravenously, the rate of administration is important because if the rate is too quick it can lead to ototoxicity. The intravenous route can be useful in acute heart failure, where the gut can become oedematous and absorption of oral furosemide may be poor. It is always worth considering the patient's ability to get to the toilet (a catheter may be needed during treatment), and adjusting the timing of diuretics so that they are not disturbed overnight (common timing is to give a dose in the morning and another just after lunch). In general, diuresis will start within an half an hour (intravenously) or an hour (oral) of dosing and will continue for 6 hours.

Furosemide tends to lower potassium levels, which should be monitored. Other electrolyte levels can fall, and it can also cause dehydration and hypotension. Elderly patients are highly susceptible to side effects that can lead to renal failure, urinary retention and falls. It is important that diuretics are not used for dependent oedema in elderly patients, but for genuine indications.

Thiazide diuretics in low doses are commonly used to lower blood pressure and are particularly effective in the elderly, although they are not now recommended as first-line agents. Bendroflumethiazide is the most common example, although indapamide (a thiazide-like diuretic) is increasingly used. Thiazides may be given in combination with other antihypertensives as a single capsule or tablet. It is important that you recognise that there are two drugs being given. Side effects are similar to loop diuretics in terms of electrolyte disturbance. In addition, they can precipitate gout and exacerbate diabetes. They will be ineffective if the glomerular filtration rate is $<30\,\mathrm{mL/min/1.73\,m^2}$.

Spironolactone is the most commonly prescribed potassium-sparing diuretic. It has experienced a resurgence as a result of recommendations for use in heart failure and resistant hypertension. It is also used in ascites and nephrotic syndrome. Spironolactone can cause hyperkalaemia and gynaecomastia/breast enlargement.

Beta blockers

Beta blockers act on the β-receptors of the autonomic nervous system, leading to a range of effects including (e.g. decrease in heart rate, decrease in blood pressure, bronchoconstriction and peripheral vasoconstriction). Some beta blockers are described as cardio-selective as they have relatively less effect on β_2-receptors;

however, this does not mean that they have no effect. Other distinctions can be made on the basis of water solubility. The more water-soluble beta blockers (including atenolol) have a reduced penetration of the blood–brain barrier, resulting in fewer central side effects (such as nightmares). A number of drugs are shorter acting but can be given as long-acting preparations.

This class of drugs is widely used for hypertension, angina, heart failure and thyrotoxicosis amongst other indications. They should be started with care at low dose and be titrated up slowly. They should not be stopped suddenly, but titrated down slowly, as there is a risk of rebound angina and hypertension.

Patients may complain of cold peripheries or tiredness, but be aware of other potentially dangerous side effects such as bradycardia and heart block, bronchospasm and hypotension.

Calcium channel blockers

Calcium channel blockers are also widely used for treating hypertension and angina. They cause vasodilation by interrupting the calcium influx into myocardial and vascular smooth muscle cells.

They can be divided into dihydropyridines (e.g. amlodipine) and non-dihydropyridines (e.g. verapamil and diltiazem). This distinction is important as indications and side effects differ. Verapamil and diltiazem are negatively inotropic and disrupt atrioventricular node conduction causing bradycardia. They should not be given in combination with beta blockers. Dihydropyridines such as amlodipine do not have these effects. Problematic side effects of dihydropyridines include headache and ankle swelling. Note that ankle swelling is not caused by oedema and does not respond particularly well to diuretic therapy. Felodipine has a number of interactions with food and other drugs.

Nitrates

Nitrates act by vasodilation, making them useful for angina. Glyceryl trinitrate (GTN) as a spray or tablet can be given to stop acute angina attacks, whereas longer-acting drugs such as isosorbide mononitrate or GTN patches have a longer anti-anginal effect. Their use can be limited by side effects such as headache and hypotension. In addition, tolerance to nitrates develops quickly. This necessitates a 'nitrate-free period' every 24 hours, which is achieved by prescribing two doses 8 hours apart (e.g. 8am and 4pm) and leaving a gap overnight or by removing the GTN patch overnight.

Intravenous GTN can be highly effective in unstable angina and severe acute heart failure under the guidance of senior medical staff. A syringe pump should be used to deliver small doses with regular blood pressure measurement. Tolerance will occur, so it is likely to be effective only in the short term.

27 Using drugs for the cardiovascular system II

Table 27.1 Cardiovascular drug classes

Drug class	Mechanism of action	Indications	Major adverse effects
ACE inhibitors/ Angiotensin II antagonists (e.g. ramipril)	Blocks production of angiotensin, thereby reducing its vasoconstrictive action	Heart failure; hypertension	Dry cough (ACE inhibitors); hypotension; hyperkalaemia; renal impairment; angio-oedema
Cardiac glycosides (e.g. digoxin)	Inhibits Na/K/ATPase increasing intracellular calcium and thereby force of myocardial contraction; stimulates vagal activity to slow conduction in AV node and bundle of His	Atrial fibrillation; heart failure	Nausea; arrhythmias/conduction disturbance
Class III anti-arrhythmics (e.g. amiodarone)	Prolongs action potential and refractory period in cardiac cells	Supraventricular and ventricular tachyarrhythmias (including atrial fibrillation)	Hepatic impairment; bradycardia; pulmonary fibrosis; hyperthyroidism or hypothyroidism; phototoxicity and skin discolouration
Adenosine	Slows conduction in the AV node by hyperpolarising cell membrane	Supraventricular tachycardia	Bronchospasm

ACE, angiotensin-converting enzyme; AV, atrioventricular

Prescribing at a Glance, First Edition. Sarah Ross. © 2014 John Wiley & Sons, Ltd. Published 2014 by John Wiley & Sons, Ltd.
Companion website: www.ataglanceseries.com/prescribing

Drugs affecting the renin–angiotensin system

Angiotensin-converting enzyme inhibitors (ACE inhibitors) and angiotensin receptor blockers (ARBs, also known as angiotensin II antagonists) interfere with the renin–angiotensin system to produce a decrease in blood pressure. They are indicated in hypertension (first-line therapy for patients under 55 years of age) and heart failure. In addition, they reduce proteinuria and are widely used in the management of diabetic nephropathy.

Unfortunately, these drugs reduce the glomerular filtration rate by about 20%, which should be manageable with normal kidneys but can be problematic in established renal impairment or older age. It is important to check renal function before starting these drugs, and again a couple of weeks into treatment to ensure there are no adverse effect. A reduction in renal function may reflect bilateral renovascular disease. ACE inhibitors and ARBs should be avoided in combination with non-steroidal anti-inflammatory drugs as the risk of renal failure is increased. Note that these drugs can have useful benefits on renal function in particular patients (e.g. those with diabetic nephropathy).

ACE inhibitors and ARBs should be started at a low dose and be titrated slowly. First-dose hypotension can be a problem, particularly if patients are taking diuretics. Other issues include: dry cough (this is caused by bradykinin and only occurs with ACE inhibitors), hyperkalaemia (particularly if given in combination with other drugs which raise potassium levels) and angioedema.

Anti-arrhythmic drugs

A range of drug classes can be used to combat arrhythmias depending on their type. Most of these agents should be started by specialists; however, in hospital settings you may be involved in acute management of common arrhythmias.

Atrial fibrillation (AF) is common and can be managed using beta blockers, digoxin (a cardiac glycoside) and non-dihydropyridine calcium channel blockers as well as amiodarone (a class III anti-arrhythmic). Digoxin is a useful drug but has a narrow therapeutic index. It has a long half-life, so if there is a need for rapid rate control in AF a loading dose regimen is needed. This is not needed if it is used for heart failure. The BNF recommends a loading dose of 0.75–1.5 mg over 24 hours. This is usually given in three divided doses, and should be reduced in elderly patients and those with reduced renal function. Unless there is a good reason not to, the oral route should be used. After that, a daily maintenance dose is given. This can be calculated using the patient's weight, but is often estimated. A digoxin level can be taken after about a week to check that the dose is appropriate. Further monitoring is not needed unless toxicity is suspected.

At toxic levels, digoxin can cause gastrointestinal upset, confusion, yellow or blurred vision, and other arrhythmias. If toxicity is suspected, a digoxin level can be taken. It may be sufficient to stop the drug; however, at very high levels the antidote (digoxin-specific antibody fragments) may be needed. Toxicity is more likely in patients who are hypokalaemic.

Adenosine is used to treat supraventricular tachycardia. This is a very short-acting drug that causes AV nodal block over a matter of seconds and should 'reset' the heart into sinus rhythm. It is usually administered in increasing doses until this occurs (up to three doses) with ECG monitoring in place. Patients should be warned that this cardioversion causes an unpleasant sensation. Adenosine should be avoided in asthmatics because of the potential for bronchospasm.

Amiodarone is a very effective drug for many arrhythmias, but is difficult to use because of its extremely long half-life and problematic side effects. It should be used under senior supervision.

28 Using drugs for the cardiovascular system III

Figure 28.1 Warfarin reversal flow chart.

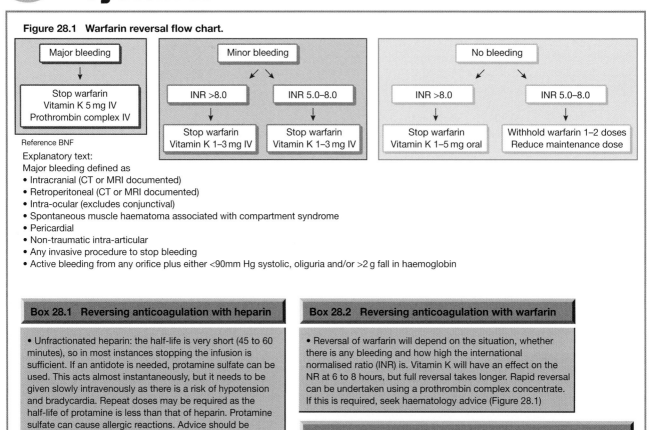

Reference BNF

Explanatory text:

Major bleeding defined as
- Intracranial (CT or MRI documented)
- Retroperitoneal (CT or MRI documented)
- Intra-ocular (excludes conjunctival)
- Spontaneous muscle haematoma associated with compartment syndrome
- Pericardial
- Non-traumatic intra-articular
- Any invasive procedure to stop bleeding
- Active bleeding from any orifice plus either <90mm Hg systolic, oliguria and/or >2 g fall in haemoglobin

---

Box 28.1 Reversing anticoagulation with heparin

- Unfractionated heparin: the half-life is very short (45 to 60 minutes), so in most instances stopping the infusion is sufficient. If an antidote is needed, protamine sulfate can be used. This acts almost instantaneously, but it needs to be given slowly intravenously as there is a risk of hypotension and bradycardia. Repeat doses may be required as the half-life of protamine is less than that of heparin. Protamine sulfate can cause allergic reactions. Advice should be sought from a haematologist.

- Low molecular weight heparin: the half-life is about 4 hours. Protamine sulfate can be used, but will only achieve partial reversal, and it is not clear how clinically effective this is.

Box 28.2 Reversing anticoagulation with warfarin

- Reversal of warfarin will depend on the situation, whether there is any bleeding and how high the international normalised ratio (INR) is. Vitamin K will have an effect on the NR at 6 to 8 hours, but full reversal takes longer. Rapid reversal can be undertaken using a prothrombin complex concentrate. If this is required, seek haematology advice (Figure 28.1)

Box 28.3 Target INR (within 0.5 of)

- INR 2.5: treatment of DVT/PE; atrial fibrillation
- INR 3.5: recurrent DVT/PE

Different tissue and metallic prosthetic valves will require different target INRs.

DVT, deep vein thrombosis; INR, international normalised ratio; PE, pulmonary embolism.

Table 28.1 Initiating and varying unfractionated heparin

aPTT ratio	Infusion rate adjustment	Recheck aPTT ratio
More than 4.00	Stop infusion for 1 hour then reduce by 500 IU (0.5 mL per hour)	After 6 hours
3.01–4.00	Reduce by 300 IU (0.3 mL per hour)	After 6 hours
2.51–3.00	Reduce by 100 IU (0.1 mL per hour)	After 6 hours
1.5 – 2.5	No change	After 6 hours
1.2–1.49	Increase by 200 IU (0.2 mL per hour)	After 6 hours
Less than 1.2	Increase by 400 IU (0.4 mL per hour)	After 6 hours

Initial intravenous bolus of 5000 units. Continuous infusion of 18 mg/kg/hr. Check the activated partial thromboplastin time (aPTT) ratio at 6 hours, then follow a protocol such as the one shown here.

Antiplatelet drugs

Antiplatelet agents are widely used for a number of indications including transient ischaemic attack/stroke, ischaemic heart disease and peripheral vascular disease. Drug examples include: aspirin, dipyridamole and clopidogrel, which work through different mechanisms to reduce platelet aggregation, and thereby have an important role in preventing clot formation on arterosclerotic plaques. This mechanism of action explains why unwanted bleeding side effects occur. Gastrointestinal haemorrhage is an important side effect to consider when prescribing these drugs, and rates are roughly similar between different drugs. Aspirin also has anti-prostaglandin actions, increasing the risk of peptic ulceration. True aspirin allergy is rare, but if present clopidogrel can be substituted. Dipyridamole has haemodynamic effects that can precipitate angina. It should be avoided in patients with heart disease.

Combinations of antiplatelet drugs have increased efficacy but also have higher risks of side effects.

Both aspirin and clopidogrel cause irreversible platelet inhibition. On cessation, continued effects are dependent on the lifespan of these platelets (about 5 days). In acute stroke or myocardial infarction, it is argued that using a higher 'loading' dose will increase the number of platelets affected. Doses of 300 mg of aspirin and clopidogrel are often used initially, followed by maintenance doses of 75 mg.

Anticoagulants

Anticoagulant drugs act on various parts of the coagulation cascade to prevent clot formation. Traditionally heparins and warfarin were the mainstay of treatment; however, newer agents are adding to therapeutic options. While the choice of anticoagulant may be a senior decision, you will need to be familiar with these drugs and the practical issues around their use including how to reverse anticoagulation (Figure 28.1, Boxes 28.1 and 28.2).

Heparin is available as low molecular weight heparin (e.g. enoxaparin). This is given as a subcutaneous injection, once or twice a day. Different doses are used for different indications, which include deep vein thrombosis (DVT) prophylaxis, treatment of DVT/pulmonary embolism (PE) and acute coronary syndromes. Doses are calculated using the patient's weight. No routine monitoring is needed. Low molecular weight heparins are less suitable in renal failure.

The other option is unfractionated heparin, which is given intravenously as a loading bolus followed by a continuous infusion, and requires regular monitoring of the activated partial thromboplastin time (aPTT) ratio to ensure the appropriate dose. Most hospitals will have a protocol to assist in decision making around dose adjustments (Table 28.1). The aPTT ratio should be rechecked 6 hours after a dose change. The advantage of unfractionated heparin is its short half-life, which means that it is highly flexible in patients who need surgical intervention or who are at high risk of bleeding. Side effects of heparin are unwanted bleeding and thrombocytopenia.

Warfarin works by inhibiting the formation of vitamin K dependent clotting factors. It is monitored by the prothrombin ratio (or INR). Different targets are used for different conditions (Box 28.3). It is given orally, and has a wide inter-patient variability that necessitates careful initial monitoring and dose selection. Daily INRs are needed until a stable dose is reached. Thereafter regular monitoring is needed. Warfarin has a very long half-life and loading doses are needed if rapid anticoagulation is needed. Protocols, including the Fennerty regimen, are available to guide prescribers (see Chapter 38). It is important to remember that changes in dose may take several days to translate into change in INR. Drug–drug and drug–food interactions are common, and it is critical that you are aware of possible under or over anticoagulation (which can be life threatening) when prescribing new drugs to patients who are taking warfarin. Antibiotics are a common culprit, but the new prescriber is wise to check the BNF for information on any new drug.

New agents (direct inhibitors of thrombin or factor Xa) are available and may be favoured over warfarin because of the lack of need for laboratory monitoring, fewer interactions and set doses.

29 Using drugs for the respiratory system

Figure 29.1 How to use a metered dose inhaler (MDI).

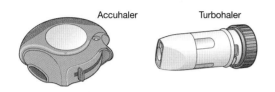

Hold the inhaler upright and shake
Remove the cap
Breathe out
Close lips around inhaler and breathe in slowly whilst pressing down on the inhaler
Hold breath for 5-10 seconds then breathe out
Wait a few seconds then repeat the above process
Replace inhaler cap

Figure 29.2 How to use a dry powder inhaler

Accuhaler   Turbohaler

Remove cap
Prime device for delivery (this varies between types)
Breathe out
Close lips around inhaler and breathe in steadily and deeply
Hold breath for 5-10 seconds
Wait a few seconds then repeat the process if a second dose is required
Replace inhaler cap

Figure 29.3 How to use a spacer.

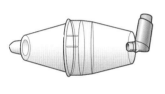

Shake the inhaler
Remove the cap from your inhaler, and from your spacer (if it has one)
Put the inhaler into the end of the spacer
Breathe out
Bring the spacer to your mouth close your lips around it (some devices have a mask to breathe through)
Press the top of your inhaler once
Take a slow controlled deep breath in and hold for 10 seconds OR take 5 slow controlled breaths in and out.

NB: A spacer is only suitable for use with an metered dose inhaler.

Box 29.1

The benefits of bronchodilator therapy can be limited by poor inhaler technique. It is vital that this is considered when prescribing, as different devices may be useful for different groups. In addition, inhaler technique should be taught. Spacer devices may be useful in children and some adults who find it difficult to use a metered dose inhaler.

Box 29.2 How to clean a spacer

Spacers should be cleaned by washing in warm water with kitchen detergent and allowing to air dry without rinsing. Drying with a cloth can result in static that can reduce the availability of dose.

Most drugs used in respiratory disease are inhaled. The benefits of bronchodilator therapy for patients can be limited by poor inhaler technique. It is vital that this is considered when prescribing, as different devices may be useful for different groups (Figures 29.1 and 29.2). In addition, inhaler technique should be taught. Spacer devices may be useful in children and some adults who find it difficult to use an MDI (Figure 29.3 and Boxes 29.1 and 29.2).

β_2-Agonists

β_2-Adrenoceptor agonists are primarily used in the management of asthma and chronic obstructive pulmonary disease (COPD). They are divided into short-acting and long-acting drugs.

Salbutamol is the most commonly used short-acting β_2-agonist prescribed for relief of acute symptoms. It is usually taken as an inhaled medicine, but it can be given by nebuliser, orally or parenterally. Nebulised salbutamol is useful in acute asthma (driven by oxygen rather than air), with parenteral routes being reserved for life-threatening attacks. In children, a metered dose inhaler (MDI) plus spacer is recommended in mild to moderate acute attacks. The oral route is very rarely used.

Long-acting β_2-agonists include salmeterol and formoterol. These drugs are used in the long-term management of asthma and COPD and are prescribed regularly. They are only available as inhalers. Their duration of action is approximately 12 hours, allowing for twice-daily dosing. Current guidelines recommend introducing a long-acting β_2-agonist as a third-line drug once regular

Prescribing at a Glance, First Edition. Sarah Ross. © 2014 John Wiley & Sons, Ltd. Published 2014 by John Wiley & Sons, Ltd.
Companion website: www.ataglanceseries.com/prescribing

low-dose corticosteroids have been tried. Ideally, they should be used for the minimum effective duration and stopped once good control of asthma has been achieved. This is because of concerns over the incidence of severe asthma attacks in patients using long-acting β_2-agonists over the long term. In addition, they should not be used without inhaled corticosteroids because of evidence of increased mortality.

Nebulised salbutamol is also used as an acute treatment for severe hyperkalaemia.

Combination inhaled preparations with corticosteroids are available and may have advantages in reducing the burden on patients and increasing compliance.

β_2-Agonists are normally well tolerated. Common side effects include tremor and tachycardia (leading to palpitations). Less commonly tachyarrhythmias can occur, and these drugs should be used cautiously in patients who are at high risk (i.e. those with cardiovascular disease and susceptibility to QT prolongation). Hypokalaemia can occur in patients where large quantities of β_2-agonist are used, and therefore potassium levels should be monitored.

Antimuscarinics

Drugs acting on muscarinic receptors within the parasympathetic nervous system have bronchodilatory effects that can be harnessed for the treatment of both asthma and COPD. Ipratropium is a short-acting drug, which is used for symptomatic relief in COPD. However, it acts less quickly than a short-acting β_2-agonist. Ipratropium can be given by both inhaler and nebuliser. The nebulised version is useful as an addition to salbutamol in acute bronchospasm.

Tiotropium is a long-acting antimuscarinic. It has been shown to reduce exacerbations of COPD. It is only available as an inhaler.

Typical antimuscarinic side effects such as dry mouth can be experienced, but other side effects should be rare with inhaled use. As with other inhalers, oral candidiasis and throat irritation can be a problem.

Theophyllines

Theophylline is a xanthine, which can be given orally or intravenously (as aminophylline that is a mix of theophylline and ethylenediamine, which makes it more soluble). It offers an additional option in the management of asthma and COPD, primarily as a fourth-line agent in chronic situations, but it can be used as treatment for acute bronchospasm. It is a challenging drug to use safely for a number of reasons, including a narrow therapeutic index and a propensity for drug–drug interactions.

Side effects include nausea and vomiting, diarrhoea, tachyarrhythmias and convulsions. Hypokalaemia is also a problem, particularly if given along with salbutamol in the acute situation.

When given orally, it should be prescribed by brand name as there are significant differences in bioavailability between brands.

Theophylline levels should be monitored during intravenous use, at 4 to 6 hours after treatment is started. A loading dose is normally given, but should be omitted if the patient has been taking an oral preparation. Dosage should be calculated by weight and adjusted according to plasma concentration. It is important that this is performed using the ideal body weight in obese patients.

Theophylline is metabolised by the hepatic cytochrome P450 system, and levels can be raised if enzyme inhibiting drugs are used. Remember that these drugs include commonly prescribed antibiotics such as clarithromycin that may be given concurrently for lung infections. Smoking may induce metabolism and reduce the efficacy of theophyllines.

Corticosteroids

Regular inhaled corticosteroids (primarily beclometasone, budesonide and fluticasone) are recommended in the British Thoracic Society asthma management guidelines for both adults and children. They can also be used in selected patients with COPD. Inhalers come in a variety of strengths, therefore the dose and number of inhalations (puffs) should be noted on all prescriptions. There does not seem to be any particular benefit of one drug over another. Inhaled steroids are also available in combination preparations with long-acting β_2-agonists. Low-dose inhaled steroids generally have fewer side effects than systemic steroids, but at higher doses systemic side effects are seen (see Chapter 34 for discussion). Oral candidiasis is very common with inhaled steroids, and this can be minimised by using a spacer and by rinsing the mouth with water after inhalation.

Oral steroids (normally prednisolone) are also used in asthma management and in exacerbations of COPD.

Leukotriene receptor antagonists

Montelukast and zafirlukast are bronchodilators that have an additive effect to other asthma therapy, particularly in exercise-induced asthma and with allergic rhinitis. They are taken orally. Current guidelines suggest that they can be used after corticosteroids and long-acting β_2-agonists have been added. Side effects include gastrointestinal disturbance and headache. Particular issues with hepatic toxicity can occur rarely with zafirlukast, and both drugs have been implicated in the development of Churg–Strauss syndrome.

Other drugs

Magnesium sulfate can be used in acute severe/life-threatening asthma as an intravenous infusion. This should only be started by senior doctors as serious adverse effects of hypotension, arrhythmias, coma and muscle weakness can occur. It also has uses in eclampsia and some arrhythmias.

Antihistamines are widely used in asthmatic patients who have an atopic component, as well as by patients with allergic rhinitis. Many drugs are available as over-the-counter preparations. Sedation is the most common side effect, and some newer agents are described as non-sedating although these are really less sedating and can still cause problems. Antimuscarinic side effects may occur and can contribute to psychomotor impairment, urinary retention and constipation, particularly in the elderly. These are less problematic with the newer agents.

Mucolytics (e.g. carbocisteine) can be used in COPD to facilitate clearance of mucous by reducing its viscosity. They should be avoided in patients with a history of peptic ulcer disease.

30 Using drugs for the neurological system I

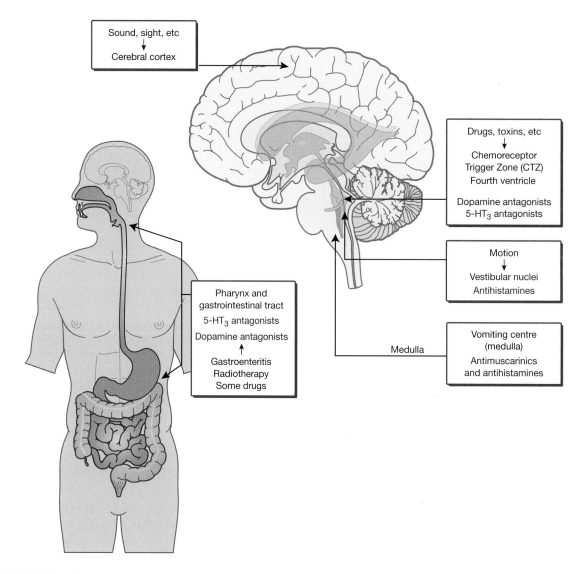

Figure 30.1 Anti-emetic sites of action. Note that stimuli are in black and the drugs that act on each area are in red.

Sound, sight, etc
↓
Cerebral cortex

Drugs, toxins, etc
↓
Chemoreceptor
Trigger Zone (CTZ)
Fourth ventricle

Dopamine antagonists
5-HT₃ antagonists

Motion
↓
Vestibular nuclei
Antihistamines

Pharynx and
gastrointestinal tract
5-HT₃ antagonists
Dopamine antagonists
↑
Gastroenteritis
Radiotherapy
Some drugs

Medulla

Vomiting centre
(medulla)
Antimuscarinics
and antihistamines

Anticonvulsants

Junior prescribers will rarely be asked to initiate anticonvulsant treatment, which should be left to a specialist; however, all doctors should be able to treat epileptic emergencies. It is also important to be aware of drug interactions and other common issues with these drugs that are taken by a large group of patients.

Benzodiazepines are first-line drugs for managing prolonged seizures. Depending on the situation, it is possible to administer these via a buccal, rectal or intravenous route. Ideally in a hospital setting, a single dose of 4 mg of lorazepam should be given intravenously. This can be repeated after 10 minutes if necessary. Diazepam may be used as an alternative but as it causes thrombophlebitis, it is a second-line choice. In situations where there is no intravenous access or resuscitation facilities are not available, buccal midazolam or rectal diazepam solutions can be given. If benzodiazepine treatment is unsuccessful, intravenous phenytoin should be administered. A loading dose is normally given by slow intravenous injection (15–20 mg/kg).

Benzodiazepines (particularly if administered by the intravenous route) can reduce the respiratory drive and cause hypotension. Intravenous phenytoin may also induce bradycardia and hypotension. The patient should therefore be closely monitored.

The continued prescription of anticonvulsants when a patient is unable to eat is important if seizures are to be avoided. Bioavailability may differ between different formulations, so care is needed in converting an oral tablet dose to a liquid (for nasogastric tube administration), an intravenous solution or a suppository. It is wise to consult a pharmacist when making these conversions.

Drug interactions are particularly common when prescribing anticonvulsants. Phenytoin and carbamazepine act as enzyme inducers, and valproate as an enzyme inhibitor. They may affect the concentration of other drugs, necessitating dose adjustments to ensure efficacy or to avoid toxicity. In addition, phenytoin can be the target of enzyme inducers/inhibitors. Newer anticonvulsants generally have fewer interactions, but it is sensible to check with a reference source before prescribing an anticonvulsant or adding a new drug for a patient taking anticonvulsants.

Anti-emetics

Nausea and vomiting are unpleasant symptoms in many illnesses. A range of anti-emetic drugs are available; however, they act in different ways and therefore a thoughtful approach to drug choice is needed.

The brain contains a 'vomiting centre' within the medulla that is linked to the pharynx/gut, the vestibular system and the chemoreceptor trigger zone. Stimulation of any of these areas can induce symptoms. Particular classes of anti-emetic dugs target particular neurotransmitters found in these areas (Figure 30.1). Antihistamines (e.g. cyclizine) act at the vomiting centre and in the vestibular nuclei. They are therefore helpful in most types of nausea, but particularly useful in raised intracranial pressure and in vestibular causes such as motion sickness. Phenothiazines (e.g. prochlorperazine) are dopamine agonists that act on dopaminergic receptors in the chemoreceptor trigger zone. These can be useful in postoperative situations, in drug induced nausea and in radiotherapy. Dopamine agonists that act peripherally in the gut are metoclopramide (which crosses the blood–brain barrier) and domperidone (which does not). These are helpful through their prokinetic actions in situations where slowed gut transit is causing symptoms, but are dangerous if the bowel is obstructed (where they can cause perforation). The 5-HT$_3$ antagonists act on the chemoreceptor trigger zone and in the gut, and are efficacious in nausea caused by chemotherapy or radiotherapy. They are also useful postoperatively.

Broad-spectrum anti-emetics (e.g. levomepromazine) are those that act on multiple receptor types.

Side effects from anti-emetics are rarely problematic; however, some important issues can occur. Extrapyramidal movements are caused by metoclopramide and the phenothiazines. Young women and the elderly seem to be more susceptible, and reactions usually stop with drug withdrawal. Patients with Parkinson's disease can experience worsening of symptoms. In these cases, domperidone may be helpful as it does not produce extrapyramidal effects. Drowsiness can be an issue with antihistamines, as can dry mouth and other anticholinergic symptoms. Constipation is a recognised side effect of antihistamines and 5-HT$_3$ antagonists, and may be unhelpful if this is already contributing to vomiting.

31 Using drugs for the neurological system II

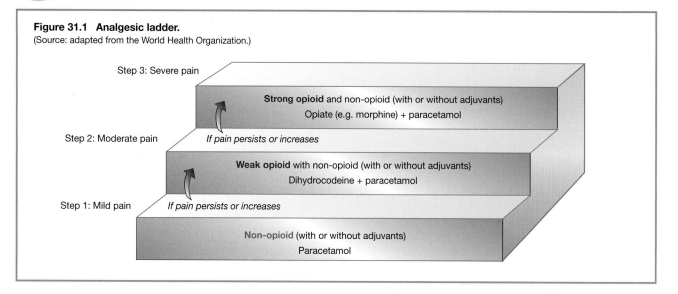

Figure 31.1 Analgesic ladder.
(Source: adapted from the World Health Organization.)

Step 3: Severe pain

Strong opioid and non-opioid (with or without adjuvants)
Opiate (e.g. morphine) + paracetamol

Step 2: Moderate pain   *If pain persists or increases*

Weak opioid with non-opioid (with or without adjuvants)
Dihydrocodeine + paracetamol

Step 1: Mild pain   *If pain persists or increases*

Non-opioid (with or without adjuvants)
Paracetamol

Analgesics

Analgesic drugs are generally divided into non-opioid (paracetamol and non-steroidal anti-inflammatory drugs [NSAIDS]) and opioid agents. Opioids are either weak (e.g. codeine) or strong (e.g. morphine). In addition, adjuvant drugs such as antidepressants and anticonvulsants can be used for particular types of pain. Pain is a common symptom, leading to widespread use of these drugs. It is therefore important to have a good understanding of how they work and when they should be used.

Paracetamol

Paracetamol is available over the counter, and is widely regarded as a safe, non-toxic drug. It is beneficial for a variety of types of pain, and has very few side effects as long as it is taken in appropriate doses. Overdose can lead to liver failure and can be accidental rather than deliberate if the patient is underweight or taking combination analgesics that contain paracetamol. Oral preparations have been available for a long time, and the relatively recent addition of an intravenous preparation has been welcome.

Non-steroidal anti-inflammatory drugs

NSAIDs are also widely used in relieving pain and reducing inflammation, but are more problematic because of adverse effects. These include gastrointestinal haemorrhage and renal impairment. Patients with asthma may experience bronchospasm with NSAIDs. It is vital that these potentially very serious adverse effects are considered before prescribing. As ever, the lowest effective dose should be prescribed for the shortest possible time to avoid unwanted effects.

Opioids

Opioid drugs act on opioid receptors. They may be naturally occurring opiates such as morphine, or synthetic opioids such as oxycodone. Efficacy and safety are similar between these groups.

Weak opioids are used for mild to moderate pain. They are relatively ineffective if prescribed alone, but have a synergistic effect with paracetamol with which they work well in combination. Strong opioids are indicated for moderate to severe pain and are 'controlled drugs' (regulated by the Misuse of Drugs Act). It is sensible to move from a weak to a strong opioid rather than combining these.

Opioids are very versatile being available for oral and parenteral use. Transcutaneous patches, intranasal sprays and buccal preparations of newer agents are available and can be beneficial for selected populations.

Start opioids at low dose and titrate upwards. Side effects are common, and toxicity is identified by myoclonus, hallucinations, drowsiness and reduced respiratory rate. Care is needed to avoid respiratory arrest. In chronic stable use, this is less problematic and other symptoms predominate; however, it is a danger when increasing doses. Constipation is a recognised unwanted effect that is normally present throughout treatment and a laxative should always be prescribed. Nausea tends to settle after the first few days, so long-term anti-emetic drugs are less commonly needed. Other side effects include drowsiness, itch and sometimes hyperaesthesia.

In general, morphine should be used as first-line therapy, with alternative opioids (such as oxycodone) reserved for use by experts in pain management or for specific patient populations. Adjuvant analgesics are also best used by experienced prescribers.

Use of analgesics is guided by the World Health Organization pain ladder (Figure 31.1), which advocates starting with paracetamol as a first step, adding a weak opioid as a second step and changing to a strong opioid as a third step, with the addition of adjuvants as needed. This is not always appropriate, for example if the patient presents with severe pain, when it is perfectly acceptable to start at the top of the ladder. Ideally, analgesics should be prescribed regularly to ensure good pain control, with 'breakthrough' additional doses as necessary. Similarly, if possible, the oral route is preferred.

When starting oral morphine for longer term use, one of the short-acting preparations such as morphine oral solution or Sevredol® should be used. This can be prescribed as required over the first 24 to 48 hours, and can be administered as often as hourly. This will give a good estimate of the total daily dose required. A longer-acting morphine such as MST continus or MXL can then be used. The dose will be half the total use over 24 hours given twice a day (MST continus) or the total dose if MXL is used. It is really important to ensure that MST continus is given at exactly 12 hour intervals, which may not line up with standard administration rounds. A 'breakthrough dose' of short-acting morphine should be prescribed in addition to the long-acting morphine. The dose should be one-sixth to one-tenth of the total daily morphine dose.

Sedatives

Hypnotics can be prescribed to aid sleep or to sedate agitated and distressed patients. They are commonly used, despite guidance that suggests they should be reserved for short-term use in severe anxiety or insomnia. Benzodiazepines and z-drugs (i.e. zopiclone and zolpidem) are the available options. Occasionally, sedating antihistamines or melatonin may also be used to induce sleep.

Confusion and delirium leading to agitation in the elderly is a common occurrence in hospital, and non-pharmacological management is preferred where possible. Adding further drugs may worsen these states and cause more harm than good. Remember that the half-life of most of these drugs is longer than the normal duration of sleep and can be prolonged in the elderly. This can lead to 'hangover' effects and can result in increased confusion and falls.

Tolerance to hypnotic drug effects occurs rapidly, and withdrawal can cause rebound insomnia. Hypnotics can also cause a degree of respiratory depression.

Alcohol withdrawal is frequently identified in hospital, and short courses of treatment with benzodiazepines are acceptable in managing withdrawal and preventing seizures. In general, the dose should be titrated using a validated scoring system and reduced fairly quickly over the first few days.

Antipsychotic drugs can be used for agitation, particularly where the patient's behaviour is a danger to themselves or others. This is often in addition to benzodiazepines. Local protocols should be followed, and reduced doses used in the elderly. Bear in mind that extrapyramidal movements, prolonged QT interval, arrhythmias and hypotension may occur along with a list of other adverse effects.

32 Using drugs for infection

> **Box 32.1 Signs of sepsis**
>
> Two or more of the following:
> - Temperature >38°C or <36°C
> - Heart rate > 90bpm
> - Respiratory rate > 20 breaths/minute
> - White cell count >12 or <4)
>
> Plus suspected or proven infection

Basic principles

Antimicrobial drugs revolutionised medicine when first discovered, but more recently their widespread use has been linked with the appearance of resistant organisms such as methicillin-resistant *Staphylococcus aureus* (MRSA) and infection with *Clostridium difficile*. You should take care when using antimicrobials and follow good practice guidance to avoid these issues.

An antimicrobial agent should only be prescribed when absolutely necessary. If needed, the selection of the drug should be based on the likely causative bacteria, virus, fungus or parasite. A good knowledge of infectious disease and the likely causes of particular clinical syndromes are required. Where possible, a clear diagnosis should be made. Samples from the potential site of infection should be sent to the microbiology laboratory for microscopy and culture, as isolating the individual infecting microbe, and testing its sensitivity to a range of possible therapies, gives the best guide for treatment. In every day practice, treatment may be required before these samples can be fully processed. This necessitates making an initial best choice based on the available information, which can later be changed according to culture and sensitivity results.

Antimicrobial drugs can be thought of as having narrow or broad-spectrum coverage, depending on the range of organisms they are effective against. It is usually best to target a single narrow spectrum agent to the likely suspected infection (for instance, trimethoprim when an urinary tract infection is suspected in women rather than a cephalosporin). At times, however, it can be helpful to use combinations (usually where the source of infection is known, such as soft tissue infection where both benzylpenicillin and flucloxacillin are used) or a broader spectrum medicine (where the source is not known).

Patterns of drug resistance vary geographically. Local guidance should be sought about the best choice of antimicrobial drug. This may be set out in an antibiotic formulary, which you should normally follow. Guidance will also be given on the duration of treatment. Here, a balance must be struck between ensuring adequate treatment to avoid recurrence of a resistant organism and the principle of using the lowest effective dose for the shortest time.

Doctors are notoriously poor at recording information about antimicrobial treatment. It is important to record a start date and intended duration (with a planned review date) in both the notes and the drug chart. In addition, the likely diagnosis and any microbiology results should be written down. Indicators of infection severity should also be noted, including temperature, pulse, blood pressure, respiratory rate, white cell count and C-reactive protein (CRP).

Consideration should be given to the route of administration. Intravenous antibiotics are overused, with implications for the patient (i.e. potential for missed doses, increased error and adverse effect rate, infection of intravenous lines) and wider resources (i.e. increased cost, staff time). This route should be reserved for severe infection or for those patients where the oral route cannot be used. Where the intravenous route is used, you should attempt to switch to the oral route early in the treatment. Intravenous antibiotics should be changed to oral if there are no signs of ongoing sepsis (Box 32.1) and if the oral route is possible. Exceptions include infections that require longer periods of intravenous therapy (e.g. endocarditis) or skin and soft tissue infection where the tissue penetration of oral antibiotics is generally poor.

Some adverse effects of antimicrobials are common to all groups. Allergy is common, particularly to penicillins and cephalosporins. This means that all patients who are prescribed antimicrobials should be asked about allergies.

C. difficile infection can be caused by any antibiotic, but some are more commonly implicated than others. Many hospitals have restricted the use of certain drugs to reduce the incidence. Antibiotic-related diarrhoea can also be caused by a range of therapies without actual *C. difficile* infection.

Some specific drugs
Penicillins and cephalosporins

Penicillins are commonly used drugs that are active against most Gram-positive organisms through inhibition of cell wall synthesis. Resistance is generally due to β-lactamase that can be overcome in many cases by giving clavulanic acid, as is present in co-amoxiclav. Allergy is found in up to 10% of patients. Cephalosporins are similar drugs and provide similar antibiotic coverage, but they have greater stability against β-lactamases. There is some crossover of allergy with penicillins, so this should be considered when prescribing and an assessment of risk should be made (based on the

Prescribing at a Glance, First Edition. Sarah Ross. © 2014 John Wiley & Sons, Ltd. Published 2014 by John Wiley & Sons, Ltd.
Companion website: www.ataglanceseries.com/prescribing

nature and timing of previous reaction and the generation of cephalosporin to be used).

Macrolides
Clarithromycin and erythromycin are commonly used antibiotics with similar effects to penicillins. In addition, they are useful in atypical pneumonia. Macrolides are hepatic enzyme inhibitors, and can cause a rise in INR when co-prescribed with warfarin, amongst other interactions.

Quinolones
These drugs (e.g. ciprofloxacin, levofloxacin) have activity against both Gram-positive and negative organisms. Use of ciprofloxacin has reduced, given its tendency to cause *C. difficile* infection. It also acts as a hepatic enzyme inhibitor.

Sulphonamides
Trimethoprim is widely used for urinary tract infection. Co-trimoxazole contains sulfamethoxazole in addition to trimethoprim. It has a broad spectrum of activity against both Gram-positive and Gram negative organisms, and has become more frequently used as penicillins and cephalopsorins have become more restricted. As they act by disrupting folate synthesis, they can inhibit bone marrow production. Stevens–Johnson syndrome, a serious hypersensitivity reaction that affects skin and mucous membranes, can occur.

Aminoglycosides
Gentamicin is the most commonly used aminoglycoside. It is a powerful but toxic drug that requires very careful use and monitoring. Gentamicin works by disrupting RNA synthesis within Gram negative organisms. It is renally excreted, but can also cause renal damage. Particular local systems for prescribing and monitoring gentamicin will be in place and should be followed.

Glycopeptide antibiotics
Vancomycin is increasingly used for the treatment of MRSA and *C. difficile* infections. When used intravenously, it has a narrow therapeutic index and requires monitoring. Renal damage and blood disorders can occur. Oral use does not require monitoring as the risks are far lower.

Antifungals
Antifungal drugs mainly act by disrupting the fungal cell membrane. Common fungal infections include *Candida* and tinea. Immunocompromised patients may also develop aspergillosis, cryptococcosis and histoplasmosis. Oral and vaginal candidasis is treated with topical treatments (nystatin, miconazole) and fluconazole. Systemic candidiasis may require more powerful therapies. Terbinafine, itraconazole and other drugs are used to combat nail and skin infections. Amphotericin is a powerful and toxic antifungal drug used in immunocompromised patients with systemic fungal infections.

Fluconazole and itraconazole can cause hepatic damage, QT interval prolongation and are liver enzyme inhibitors. Amphotericin is normally given as an intravenous lipid formulation, as this is less toxic. It should be used only by senior experienced clinicians. Problems with renal impairment, hypokalaemia and hypomagnesaemia, arrhythmias, anaemia, neurological side effects and hepatic injury are seen.

Antivirals
A range of antiretroviral drugs targeted at human immunodeficiency virus (HIV) infection are in use that act on various targets in the HIV viral cell. While these should be started by a specialist in infectious disease, patients will sometimes be seen by other doctors. Antiretrovirals are toxic, causing problems such as lipodystrophy, hepatic impairment, lactic acidosis, osteonecrosis, bone marrow suppression, hypersensitivity reactions and hyperglycaemia. They are always given in combination and should not be stopped without discussion with a senior doctor.

Aciclovir is widely used to treat herpes simplex and zoster infections. It acts against DNA polymerases in viral cells. It can be given orally or parenterally, but has a short half-life, necessitating frequent administration. Doses vary by indication, and should be reduced in renal impairment.

33 Using drugs for the endocrine system I

Table 33.1   Insulin types

Type	Name
Short acting	Actrapid® Humalog® (insulin lispro) Humulin® S NovoRapid® (insulin aspart)
Biphasic	Humalog® mix 25 Humalog® mix 50 Humulin® M3 NovoMix 30
Intermediate acting	Humulin® I Insulatard®
Long acting	Lantus® (insulin glargine) Levemir® (insulin detemir)

Figure 33.1   Timing of insulin effects.

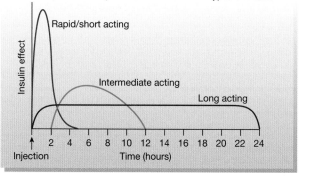

Comparison of equal amounts of different types of insulin

Common insulin regimes

Figure 33.2   Basal bonus.

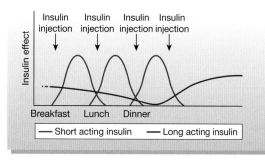

Figure 33.3   Twice-daily biphasic regimen.

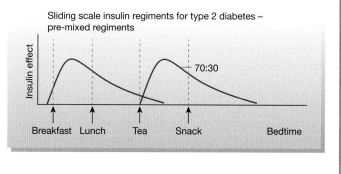

Sliding scale insulin regiments for type 2 diabetes – pre-mixed regiments

Prescribing at a Glance, First Edition. Sarah Ross. © 2014 John Wiley & Sons, Ltd. Published 2014 by John Wiley & Sons, Ltd.

Companion website: www.ataglanceseries.com/prescribing

Insulins

Insulins are widely used for the treatment of all types of diabetes mellitus as well as for the emergency treatment of hyperkalaemia. There are many different preparations, which can be confusing for prescribers, and errors are common. It is critical that you understand the types of insulin and the regimens used. It is unlikely that you will be starting or changing insulins; however, diabetes is very common and you will often be involved in continuing to prescribe insulin for hospital patients and tackling problems that may arise.

Types of insulin

Insulin is derived from humans and animals (particularly pigs). These preparations are not interchangeable. They can be divided into rapid, short, intermediate and long acting, but can also be combined into mixed preparations (Figure 33.1 and Table 33.1).

Rapid or short-acting insulins include: soluble insulin (e.g. Actrapid') and the insulin analogues insulin aspart, insulin glulisine and insulin lispro. These start acting quickly, but have a short duration of action. Soluble insulin (Actrapid') is used for continuous insulin infusions. It is widely used in hospital for diabetic patients who are acutely unwell, going for surgery or who are not able to eat. It should be given with appropriate intravenous fluids. Local protocols are often available to assist prescribers with this.

Intermediate-acting insulins include isophane insulins (also known as neutral protamine hagedorn or NPH). Long-acting insulins are insulin glargine and insulin determir.

Mixtures of short- and long-acting insulin can be used, and are referred to as biphasic insulins (i.e. they have two peaks of action). Different preparations have different proportions of short- and long-acting insulins, denoted by the term 'mix'. The number following the word 'mix' indicates the percentage of short-acting insulin (e.g. 25% in Humalog' mix 25).

Insulin names are very similar and it is vital that they are prescribed accurately. The effect of short-acting Humalog® is very different from that of biphasic Humalog' mix 25!

Insulin regimens

Typical regimens (Figures 33.2 and 33.3) are as follows:
• Once-daily long-acting insulin at night (suitable for type 2 patients only)
• Twice-daily biphasic insulin
• Basal bolus with intermediate- or long-acting insulin once a day (at night) plus short-acting insulin at each meal
• Continuous insulin infusion in an insulin pump (using short-acting insulin).

Insulins are usually administered subcutaneously, and a wide range of devices are available for patients to use. The site of injection should be varied to reduce lipodystrophy.

Patients are encouraged to monitor their blood glucose levels. Some may vary their insulin dose against these, or by 'carbohydrate counting'. Glucose levels should also be monitored closely in hospital. It is important to remember that illness can change the patient's insulin requirements. Patients with type 1 diabetes should always have some insulin prescribed, even when fasting (where a concurrent glucose infusion will be needed).

Insulin infusions

You will be asked to prescribe intravenous insulin infusions for the treatment of diabetic emergencies (i.e. diabetic ketoacidosis and hyperosmolar non-ketotic coma) or in selected patients who are not eating normally. These are standard short-acting insulin infusions where the rate of infusion is varied according to the blood glucose level. Local protocols will be available for the treatment of emergencies. Separate instructions for non-emergency insulin infusions may be available. One particularly common situation will be prescribing for a patient who is going for surgery. A general guide would be to give the patient their normal insulin the night before, to start a sliding scale insulin infusion along with glucose and potassium on the morning of surgery, and to switch back to the patient's normal regimen when they are able to eat and drink (e.g. give normal insulin before a meal, eat then stop the infusion 30 minutes later) (see Chapter 37).

Hypoglycaemia

The main adverse effect of insulin is hypoglycaemia. This can be life threatening, and patients do not always experience symptoms. It is vital that rapid treatment of hypoglycaemia is available in hospital. It is likely that there will be a local protocol that should be followed. Generally this will recommend consumption of carbohydrate if the patient is able, or using a buccal sugar preparation (such as Glucogel'). If the patient is unconscious, intravenous glucose can be given (e.g. 100 mL of 10% glucose solution) or glucagon can be administered by the subcutaneous, intramuscular or intravenous route.

Other antidiabetic drugs

Sulphonylureas

Examples of sulphonylureas are glipizide and gliclazide. These are commonly used in type 2 diabetes. They act by increasing insulin secretion from the pancreas. This means that they can cause hypoglycaemia. Weight gain can be troublesome, and so this class of drugs is usually reserved for patients who are not overweight. Both hepatic and renal impairment can cause excess hypoglycaemia, so care should be taken in patients with these problems. Other side effects include gastrointestinal upset and, rarely, hepatotoxicity.

Biguanides

Metformin is the only available biguanide. It acts by reducing hepatic gluconeogenesis and by increasing peripheral glucose use. In most instances it does not cause hypoglycaemia. It is widely used in patients with type 2 diabetes who are overweight. The main adverse effect is diarrhoea, which can be highly problematic for patients particularly at higher doses. Metformin can also cause lactic acidosis in rare cases. As this is more likely in patients with renal impairment, it should be avoided in these patients as well as those undergoing investigations that involve radiocontrast agents.

Other agents

A range of other antidiabetic agents are now available for type 2 diabetes. These include thiazolidinediones or glitazones (e.g. pioglitazone), incretin mimetics (e.g. exenatide) and DPP-4 inhibitors or gliptins (e.g. sitagliptin). These should be initiated by specialists. A number of issues with these relatively new classes of drugs have arisen, including heart failure with glitazones and pancreatitis with incretin mimetics and DPP-4 inhibitors. Other more common adverse effects include gastrointestinal upset. Remember that these drugs can cause hypoglycaemia.

Using drugs for the endocrine system II

Box 34.1 Equivalent doses of corticosteroids

Prednisolone 5 mg:

- Is equivalent to betamethasone 750 micrograms
- Is equivalent to dexamethasone 750 micrograms
- Is equivalent to hydrocortisone 20 mg
- Is equivalent to methylprednisolone 4 mg

Prescribing at a Glance, First Edition. Sarah Ross. © 2014 John Wiley & Sons, Ltd. Published 2014 by John Wiley & Sons, Ltd.

Companion website: www.ataglanceseries.com/prescribing

Corticosteroids

Corticosteroids are widely used in medicine for a range of inflammatory and malignant conditions. They can be given by almost every possible route of administration, with different drugs used for different indications and routes (Box 34.1). While topical and local application should limit systemic side effects, these do occur. Unwanted effects may vary with the length of use. There are a wide range of adverse effects, which include:

* Cushingoid features including weight gain
* Osteoporosis
* Ischaemic necrosis of femoral head
* Cataract
* Acute glaucoma
* Increased susceptibility to infection, particularly tuberculosis, varicella and *Candida*
* Hyperglycaemia
* Hypertension
* Fluid retention and worsening of heart failure
* Hypokalaemia
* Mental disturbance including psychosis.

For this reason, the minimum effective dose should be used for the shortest duration. Oral steroids are best taken in the morning to match the body's normal diurnal variation; it can cause insomnia if given late in the day.

Patients prescribed long-term corticosteroids (more than 3 weeks) should be provided with a 'steroid card' and warned not to stop their medication suddenly. In instances where oral or parenteral corticosteroids are used continually for more than 3 weeks, or in multiple short courses or at very high doses, patients should be given a reducing regimen (i.e. reduce the dose every few days until reaching 7.5 mg after which a slower reduction may be needed). This is because endogenous production of steroids will be suppressed and therefore patients may experience an Addisonian crisis without exogenous steroids. Remember that stopping inhaled steroids, especially high-dose regimens, can cause this effect. Problems may also occur in patients taking steroids (or who have recently discontinued them) who experience acute illness or trauma that will increase the body's steroid requirement. It is common practice to double the dose of any corticosteroid prescribed if this occurs. It may be necessary to give this intravenously as hydrocortisone if the patient is 'nil by mouth'.

Drugs in thyroid disease

Thyroid disease is common, and therefore some familiarity with treatments is useful. Hypothyroidism is treated almost exclusively with levothyroxine, which replenishes thyroxine levels. It should be started with care, particularly in older patients and those with cardiac disease. Liothyronine may be used by severe hypothyroidism and in hypothyroid coma by endocrinologists.

Levothyroxine is given by mouth, at a starting dose of 50 micrograms (25 micrograms in the elderly) and the dose titrated upwards over weeks until satisfactory thyroxine and thyroid stimulating hormone levels are reached. Side effects are those of hyperthyroidism, and normally due to over-treatment. It is worth remembering that thyroid function tests can be inaccurate in acute illness.

Hyperthyroidism is treated with drugs or with radio-iodine. The most commonly used medication is carbimazole, which interferes with thyroid hormone production. It is rarely initiated by non-specialists. This is a toxic drug, with bone marrow suppression being a major concern. Patients should be warned to report any incidents of a sore throat. Be wary of infection as a cause of symptoms in any unwell patient who is taking carbimazole. It should be stopped if neutropenia occurs. Co-prescription of propranolol can be useful in reducing symptoms, particularly from tachycardias.

Oral contraceptives and hormone replacement therapy

Oral contraceptives are widely used. These either contain oestrogen and progesterone (combined oral contraceptives) or progesterone alone (progesterone only contraceptives). Oral, transdermal and intrauterine options are available for the combined pill. The combined pill is usually taken for 21 days, and then stopped to allow normal menstrual bleeding. It can also be taken continuously for various indications. Drug interactions, missed doses and vomiting/diarrhoea can cause pill failure, and advice to use alternative forms of contraception should be given. Check the *British National Formulary* (BNF) for advice if this occurs. Important drug interactions occur with hepatic enzyme inducers such as anticonvulsants. It is no longer thought that antibiotics are problematic unless they induce vomiting or diarrhoea, with the exception of rifampicin. Again it is important to consult the BNF for advice on what to do if these drugs are co-prescribed.

Side effects include headache, hypertension, depression, breast changes and hepatic dysfunction. Drugs should be stopped if symptoms suggestive of major cardiac, respiratory, hepatic or neurological disease occur. Patients with a past history of venous thromboembolism, cardiac disease, migraine, stroke and breast cancer should normally not be prescribed the combined oral contraceptive pill.

Both contraceptives and hormone replacement therapy are associated with an increased risk of venous thromboembolism. When commencing these, other risk factors such as age, smoking and obesity should be considered. They should normally be stopped several weeks before major surgery to reduce the risk of postoperative deep vein thrombosis.

The combined pill is also associated with an increased risk of breast cancer and cervical cancer, although this is very low.

Progesterone only contraceptives have fewer risks and side effects, but are less effective. In general, they can be used where combined contraception is not advised.

Hormone replacement therapy is used to reduce menopausal symptoms. The choice of combined oestrogen- and progesterone-containing preparations versus those with just oestrogen is based on whether the patient still has her uterus or not (if not, oestrogen alone can be used). It carries similar (but increased) risks to the oral contraceptive pill, and additionally increases the risks of ovarian and endometrial cancers.

35 How to use drugs for the musculoskeletal system

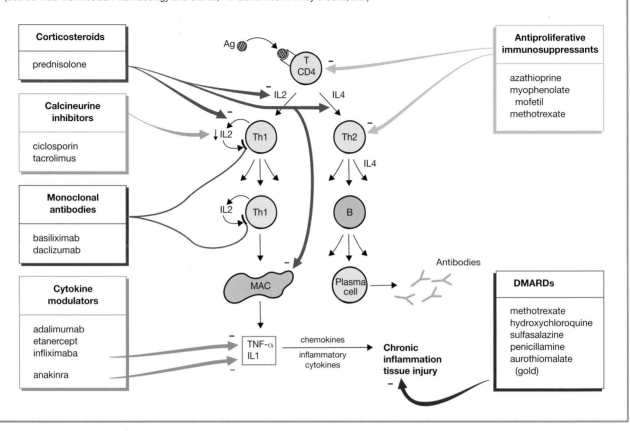

Figure 35.1 Immunosuppressants and antirheumatoid drugs.
(Source: Neal MJ. *Medical Pharmacology at a Glance,* 7th Edition. John Wiley & Sons, Ltd.)

Non-steroidal anti-inflammatories (NSAIDs)

These drugs are widely used as analgesics; however, they also have useful anti-inflammatory actions that make them popular choices in rheumatological and musculoskeletal illness. By blocking cyclo-oxygenase, prostaglandin production is reduced, attenuating the inflammatory response, thereby giving relief from swelling and stiffness. However, NSAIDs do not have any disease-modifying effects in rheumatological diseases.

Analgesic and antipyretic effects occur through the same mechanism (for further discussion of analgesia see Chapter 31).

Cyclo-oxygenase has two isoforms, COX-1 and COX-2, and selective COX-2 inhibitors such as celecoxib are available. These have similar properties to non-selective NSAIDs, but their side-effect profiles are problematic, meaning there is little advantage in using them.

NSAIDs are usually given orally, but can be given topically, rectally and parenterally. Higher doses may be used for anti-inflammatory effects than for standard analgesic effects.

NSAID use is limited by their side effects, primarily gastrointestinal (GI) haemorrhage and renal impairment. Both these prob-lems are caused by disruption of prostaglandin synthesis. It is worth noting that GI effects are not caused by local effects on the gastric mucosa, but rather systemic effects on prostaglandins, and so using parenteral routes of administration will not reduce side effects. Using a drug such as a proton pump inhibitor along with an NSAID may reduce the risk of GI bleeding. Bronchospasm can occur with NSAIDs due to increased leucotrienes, and are relatively contraindicated in patients with asthma. NSAIDs are also associated with salt and water retention in the kidneys, which may increase blood pressure and worsen heart failure. COX-2 inhibitors and diclofenac have been particularly associated with increased cardiovascular events. All these potentially very serious adverse effects must be considered before prescribing, and the lowest dose should be used for the shortest possible time.

Co-prescription of antiplatelets and/or anticoagulants with NSAIDs increases the risk of GI bleeding.

Disease-modifying antirheumatic drugs

Drugs that suppress the immune system can slow the progression of rheumatoid arthritis and other rheumatological and inflammatory diseases. These should be started and monitored by specialists, but may be encountered relatively frequently by other prescribers. They have serious adverse effects, and it is important to be aware of them; however, making changes to prescriptions should only be undertaken with senior advice.

Drugs used in musculoskeletal diseases include methotrexate, sulfasalazine, gold, penicillamine, azathioprine, mycophenolate mofetil, leflunomide and hydroxychloroquine. More recently a range of monoclonal antibodies (also known as biologics) that modulate individual cytokines have become available including, adalimumab, etanercept, infliximab and anakinra.

In simple terms, some of these drugs reduce the production of rapidly dividing cells such as lymphocytes in response to an immune stimulus by interfering with DNA synthesis (azathioprine, mycophenolate mofetil) or folate synthesis (methotrexate). Others work by inhibiting cytokines such as tumour necrosis factor alpha (adalimumab, etanercept, infliximab) and interleukin-1 (anakinra), which are produced by inflammatory cells and increase the inflammatory response. Others such as penicillamine, gold and sulfasalazine work by unknown mechanisms (Figure 35.1).

Biologics are normally given by periodic infusion. The other drugs are given in a variety of oral and parenteral routes daily, weekly or less often. This variety can lead to error, so it is important to check that the correct frequency is prescribed.

Side effects are problematic with these drugs. Patients are more susceptible to infection due to immunosuppression. Bone marrow suppression, with neutropenia, anaemia and thrombocytopenia is seen, and patients should be warned to seek medical attention if they experience potential signs such as fever, sore throat, bruising or bleeding. In addition, gold and penicillamine can cause renal damage and serious skin rashes amongst other side effects. Careful monitoring of these treatments is required, usually with regular blood tests depending on the drug used. For patients acutely admitted to hospital unwell, adverse effects should be considered as the cause of new symptoms and signs, bloods should be checked for signs of renal, liver and bone marrow abnormalities and consideration should be given to withholding these treatments.

Drugs for gout

NSAIDs, corticosteroids and colchicine are all used in the acute treatment of gout, depending on other patient factors. NSAIDs are suitable if there are no contraindications or drug interactions. Colchicine is an alternative that works by inhibiting phagocytic activity and migration of leucocytes to areas of increased uric acid, thereby reducing the inflammatory response. It can cause GI upset, and is toxic at higher doses (causing GI haemorrhage, hepatic and renal damage). Corticosteroids are an effective treatment if these treatments are not suitable.

Long-term prevention of gout can be achieved with allopurinol, which acts by inhibiting xanthine oxidase to reduce overall uric acid production. It can precipitate an attack of gout, however, or make one worse, so it should not be started during an acute episode. When initiating treatment, NSAIDs or colchicine can be used in addition to prevent this occurring. Allopurinol should be given along with an adequate fluid intake as crystallisation of urate in the urine can occur. Administration is oral, with a starting dose of 100 micrograms that can be titrated up, but should be kept at this level in renal impairment. A severe hypersensitivity reaction can occur, so allopurinol should be withdrawn if a rash occurs. Otherwise, the main adverse effects are GI.

Bisphosphonates

Bisphosphonates are widely used for the prevention of osteoporosis and for the prevention of fractures in patients with established osteoporosis. They are also used in the treatment of hypercalcaemia and in the treatment of bony metastases in breast cancer.

They act by disrupting osteoclastic bone resorption. In osteoporosis, they are given orally and can be given daily, weekly or monthly depending on the drug and preparation. This means that confusion over doses (which are often different for different frequencies) and frequency is a potential cause of error and care should be taken to ensure the correct regimen is prescribed.

In hypercalcaemia, bisphosphonates are given by intravenous infusion, and preceded by adequate hydration with 0.9% sodium chloride. In breast cancer, oral and intravenous regimens are prescribed.

Several problems with bisphosphonates are recognised. Oesophageal irritation, ulceration and strictures can occur and particular instructions are given for oral administration. Patients should be advised to take their tablet standing or sitting upright, and should remain so for at least 30 minutes. Tablets should be swallowed whole. For good absorption, they should be taken on an empty stomach and not at the same time as any other medicine. In addition, milk and calcium- containing products should be avoided for several hours. Patients should be warned to stop taking their medicine and seek medical attention if heartburn, difficulty swallowing or pain occurs. It is usually wise to avoid co-prescription of NSAIDs or other drugs that can cause GI ulceration.

Osteonecrosis of the jaw is a serious complication, tending to occur more often with intravenous bisphosphonate treatment in cancer patients than in oral treatment for osteoporosis. To reduce the risk, patients should have a dental check-up and any necessary treatment should be completed before a bisphosphonate is started. Good oral hygiene during treatment is also important.

Atypical femoral fractures can also occur rarely in patients receiving long-term therapy (5 years or more).

36 Using drugs in haematology and oncology

Table 36.1 Immunosuppression with chemotherapeutic agents

Drug	Amount of suppression	Time to nadie (from each dose)	Time to recovery (from dosing)
Alkylating agents			
Cyclophosphamide	++	10–14 days	2–4 weeks
Melphalan	++	8–10 days	5–7 weeks
Anthracyclines			
Doxorubicin	+++	10-14 days	3-4 weeks
Anti-metabolities			
Methotrexate	++ to +++	1-2 weeks	2-3 weeks
Capecitabine	+ to ++	10-14 days	2-3 weeks
Vinca alkaloids			
Etoposide	+++	1–2 weeks	2-3 weeks
Vincristine	+	7-10 days	3 weeks
Platinum compounds			
Cisplatin	++	2-3 weeks	4-6 weeks

Anaemia

Iron deficiency anaemia

Oral iron is available in several forms, but ferrous sulfate and ferrous fumarate are the most widely used. Parenteral iron is rarely used, but may be needed for some patients (e.g. renal dialysis patients). Iron supplementation is commonly prescribed at a dose of 200 mg ferrous sulfate three times a day. This should cause a normalisation of haemoglobin concentration after approximately 1 month, but should be continued for a further 3 months to replenish iron stores. Adverse effects are often seen. Nausea tends to be dose related, and therefore iron may be more tolerable if given at a lower dose. Constipation often occurs and does not seem to be dose related. Some patients experience diarrhoea instead. Patients should be warned that stool colour will change and that 'black stools' with iron is usually not a cause for concern. Side effects are similar between preparations, and combination or slow-release formulations rarely add benefit.

Megaloblastic anaemia

Vitamin B_{12} and folate deficiency can cause megaloblastic anaemia. Either or both may be required for treatment. It is important that blood transfusion is not used in these patients as it is associated with increased morbidity and mortality.

B_{12} should be supplemented parenterally (intramuscular hydroxocobalamin) as most cases of deficiency are caused by malabsorption. In most patients, an initial course of several doses of vitamin B_{12} is given over the first couple of weeks (see British National Formulary [BNF] for directions), and then prescribed 3-monthly for long-term maintenance.

Folic acid can be given orally at a dose of 5 mg per day until the anaemia is corrected (approximately 4 months). Long-term use is rarely needed. It is also used to prevent neural tube defects in pregnancy. Women at low risk of neural tube defect should take a lower dose (400 mg) prior to conception and until week 12 of pregnancy. Women at high risk (family history, previous incidence, diabetes and those taking anticonvulsant medication) should take 5 mg throughout pregnancy. These patients will normally be identified by antenatal services.

Cytotoxic drugs

Chemotherapy regimens should never be prescribed by non-specialist prescribers; however, patients with ongoing cancer therapy may present to other services with a variety of problems and therefore knowledge of generic problems can be useful.

Common problems include nausea and vomiting, gastrointestinal mucositis, bone marrow suppression, alopecia, hyperuricaemia and tumour lysis syndrome. These occur with all cytotoxic drugs but in varying ways. Nausea and vomiting should be considered at the time of chemotherapy administration and specialists will normally prescribe concurrent anti-emetic drugs. Chemotherapeutic drugs are usually divided into mild, moderate and highly emetogenic, and this can be used to predict what anti-emetics will be required. Anti-emetic prescribing is discussed in Chapter 30. The 5-HT_3 agonists and dopamine antagonists are used first line, and a range of other drugs, particularly broad-spectrum anti-emetics may also be used. Intravenous fluids may be required, particularly in patients treated with nephrotoxic agents.

Symptoms of oral mucositis may be reduced with various preparations such as Gelclair˙. Remember that candidal and herpes infections may exacerbate symptoms. Mucositis can also present as life-threatening diarrhoea, and careful fluid balance management is essential. Loperamide can be used to reduce the frequency of diarrhoea. If mucositis is caused by folate antagonists (e.g. methotrexate or fluorouracil), folinic acid can be used to reduce symptoms.

Bone marrow suppression can manifest as anaemia, immunosuppression or bleeding. This may be treated with human granulocyte colony stimulating factor (again this is normally prescribed by specialists), or transfusion of blood and platelets. Hospitals will have guidance on the antibiotics that should be used in neutropenic sepsis. Junior doctors should be alert to this possibility in all patients undergoing chemotherapy who may present to a variety of specialities. The nadir (lowest neutrophil count) usually occurs 7 to 10 days following treatment; however, cell counts can be low at any time (Table 36.1) so a high index of suspicion is needed. Rapid treatment of infection with appropriate intravenous antibiotics and fluid resuscitation is essential. Fever may be the only presenting symptom, and the source may not be obvious; remember line sepsis as a cause in patients with a central line.

Hyperuricaemia and tumour lysis syndrome should be considered as a possible complication in patients undergoing treatment for haematological malignancy, and pretreatment with allopurinol should be given along with an adequate fluid intake to prevent acute renal failure.

Specific anticancer therapies are associated with specific common adverse effects:

• Alkylating agents (e.g. cyclophosphamide, melphalan) work by disrupting cell replication through effects on DNA. Bone marrow suppression is likely, and additional issues with cystitis and pulmonary fibrosis can be seen with different agents.
• Anthracyclines (e.g. doxorubicin) are associated with cardiac toxicity and red discolouration of urine. Skin reactions also occur.
• Antimetabolites (e.g. methotrexate, capecitabine) act on folate synthesis to reduce purine and pyrimidine synthesis for DNA replication. Bone marrow suppression and mucositis are therefore commonly seen.
• Vinca alkaloids (e.g. etoposide, vincristine) are particularly known for neurotoxicity. They are also more likely to cause tissue damage if extravasation occurs. Myelosuppression is rare with vincristine, but problematic with other alkaloids.

• Platinum compounds (e.g. cisplatin) can cause nephrotoxicity, neurotoxicity and ototoxicity.

Biologics

Many newer cancer treatments are biologics targeted at a range of cell targets such as tyrosine kinase. They do not have the typical adverse effect profile of other cancer drugs, and as with all new drugs, side effects are still being discovered. The BNF and Schedule of Product Characteristics will list common problems.

Hormones in cancer treatment

Some cancers can be treated by targeting sex hormones. Oestrogens are useful in prostate cancer as are drugs such as gonadotropin-releasing hormone antagonists, which act by reducing androgens. 'Tumour flare' can be a problem within the first month of treatment with increased bone pain, ureteric obstruction and even cord compression. Following this, side effects are related to androgen depletion. Cardiac complications can also occur.

Aromatase inhibitors (e.g. tamoxifen, letrozole), widely used in breast cancer, reduce the conversion of androgens to oestrogens. As patients may be taking these drugs for many years, their effects will be commonly seen. Possible issues worth considering include increased thromboembolism risk with tamoxifen, which should be considered during any hospital stay, and gynaecological side effects.

Other drugs

Malignant hypercalcaemia is a common oncological emergency, which should be treated with intravenous saline followed by intravenous bisphosphonates (see Chapter 35).

Corticosteroids (often dexamethasone) are frequently used by cancer patients for indications such as anorexia, nausea, pain, raised intracranial pressure, gastrointestinal obstruction, spinal cord compression and superior vena cava obstruction. As high doses tend to be used, side effects are common (see Chapter 34). Proton pump inhibitors are normally co-prescribed to reduce the risk of gastrointestinal haemorrhage.

37 Using drugs in anaesthesia

Figure 37.1 Using antiplatelet and anticoagulant drugs perioperatively.
(Source: Korte W, Cattaneo M, Chassot PG, et al (2011). Peri-operative management of antiplatelet therapy in patients with coronary artery disease. Thromb Haemost 105: 743-9. Reproduced with permission from Haemostasis in Critical Care.)

Minor surgery: do not stop antiplatelet therapy

Implement multidisciplinary consult in patients with (potential) bleeding complications
Low molecular weight heparin: NOT a substitute for platelet inhibiting drugs
Avoid plasmatic anticoagulation (LMWH, OAC) during surgery

Major surgery and how to proceed		Exception	How to proceed with exception
Aspirin for primary prevention*	Stop aspirin 5 days before surgery*		
Aspirin in high-risk patients* (diabetes, history of CV events, documented CV disease, increased global risk)	Continue aspirin*	Surgery in closed space, expected major bleeding complications	• Stop aspirin 5 days before surgery* • Consider restarting within 24h*
Aspirin **plus** clopidogrel in high risk patients	1. Elective surgery: delay until no dual inhibition necessary 2. Semi-urgent surgery: continue aspirin ± clopidogrel on a case by case basis 3. Urgent surgery (within 24 hours): continue aspirin and clopidogrel	Surgery in closed space, expected major bleeding complications	*If delaying surgery not possible/ semi-urgent surgery necessary:* • Stop clopidogrel 5 days before surgery, consider bridging (short acting GPIIb/IIIa antagonist) • Consider stopping also aspirin in particular patients • Consider resuming dual antiplatelet therapy asap

Table 37.1 Properties of local anaesthetics

Drug	Onset	Maximum dose (with epinephrine)	Duration
Lidocaine	Rapid	3 mg/kg (7 mg/kg)	2 hours (4 hours)
Bupivacaine	Slow	2 mg/kg (2.5 mg/kg)	4 hours (8 hours)
Prilocaine	Medium	6 mg/kg (9 mg/kg)	1.5 hours (6 hours)

• Extends also to patients on clopidogrel monotherapy

Issues with general anaesthetics
Prescription of regular medicines preoperatively
New prescribers looking after surgical patients will need to make decisions about which medications are to be given prior to procedures and operations. Most medicines should be given normally and not omitted just because the patient is fasting, which can be a common mistake. Clear fluids along with medicines are safe up to 2 hours pre-surgery. It is important to remember that some medicines have adverse withdrawal effects that are best avoided in combination with surgery. There are, however, a number of drugs that should be withheld because of potentially adverse effects associated with perioperative use.

Antiplatelet and anticoagulant drugs pose a bleeding risk, but this must be weighed against the significant risk of myocardial infarction, stroke and other embolic events if they are stopped even briefly. Surgical teams may use particular local guidelines; however, each patient should be considered individually. In general, patients who are prescribed an antiplatelet for primary prevention of cardiovascular disease should have it stopped 5 to 7 days preoperatively. For those with proven cardiovascular disease, monotherapy with one antiplatelet should be continued with surgery; dual antiplatelet therapy with aspirin and clopidogrel is not advised unless patients have recently undergone coronary artery stenting. For patients undergoing particularly high-risk procedures where surgery is in a confined space (e.g. neurosurgery)

Prescribing at a Glance, First Edition. Sarah Ross. © 2014 John Wiley & Sons, Ltd. Published 2014 by John Wiley & Sons, Ltd.
Companion website: www.ataglanceseries.com/prescribing

or those likely to bleed significantly, all antiplatelet drugs should be stopped. For patients with coronary stents, elective surgery should be postponed until after the planned end date for dual antiplatelet therapy if possible, and expert advice sought about stopping them prematurely. Senior clinicians should be involved in decision making for these patients.

Patients on warfarin can have this stopped or converted to unfractionated heparin, which is more controllable over the perioperative period. Consider the reason for anticoagulation to determine the risks. Anticoagulation is important to continue in high-risk conditions such as metallic mitral value replacement, but may be stopped in those at lower risk (primary prevention of stroke in patients with atrial fibrillation and few other risk factors). Again this is a senior decision that should be made when planning for elective surgery. In general, warfarin can be started at the same dose as prior to surgery rather than requiring a loading dose regimen, but it is important to consider the benefits and risk to the individual patient and the speed at which anticoagulation should be re-established. In emergency cases, the anaesthetist and surgeon should decide on timing of medicines and any plan to reverse anticoagulation.

It is important that antihypertensives and rate controlling medicines such as beta blockers are continued perioperatively to ensure that heart rate and blood pressure are maintained within safe limits for anaesthesia and surgery. Omission is a common reason for cancelled surgery. Some agents, particularly angiotensin-converting enzyme inhibitors and angiotensin II antagonists should be withheld on the day of surgery because of the risk of renal impairment.

Patients taking long-term corticosteroids will need an increase in dose in the perioperative period, and are often given intravenous hydrocortisone rather than oral prednisolone.

Patients with diabetes require careful perioperative management to ensure that blood glucose levels are maintained. For patients with type I diabetes, continuous variable rate intravenous insulin is required and it is unsafe to stop insulin at any point. This will require the co-administration of glucose. It is likely that hospitals will have standard regimens that should be used for these patients. Once the patient is eating and drinking normally, their usual insulin regimen can be restarted. It is common practice to give subcutaneous insulin before a main meal and stop the intravenous infusion after eating.

Patients with type II diabetes do not have an absolute need for insulin and can be managed without an intravenous variable rate infusion in some instances. Metformin should be stopped prior to surgery as there is an increased risk of lactic acidosis. Sulphonylureas are usually withheld also. If necessary, a variable rate intravenous insulin infusion can be used to control blood glucose around the time of the operation.

Anticonvulsants should be continued perioperatively, and if necessary patients taking drugs that are not available in a parenteral formulation may be given intravenous phenytoin instead. This should be discussed with the anaesthetist.

Given their side effects, it is usually wise to withhold non-steroidal anti-inflammatory drugs for a few days prior to surgery.

Prophylaxis of thromboembolism

Major surgery increases the risk of deep venous thrombosis and pulmonary embolism substantially so it is important that prophylactic therapy is considered. This will usually be low molecular weight heparin at lower dose than the standard treatment dose (listed in the *British National Formulary*) although fondaparinux is also an option. Surgical units will generally have their own policy that should be followed.

Complications following general anaesthesia

It is important to remember that a range of drugs may be used in the anaesthetic setting beyond general anaesthetics and muscle relaxants, including anxiolytics (benzodiazepines), analgesics, anti-emetics, acid suppressing and antibiotics. These all have adverse effects that may manifest after the operation. In particular, sedation, respiratory depression, cardiac depression, nausea and vomiting, and hepatotoxicity may be problematic.

Local anaesthetics

A number of local anaesthetics are available, but lidocaine (lignocaine) is the most widely used. They act by inactivating sodium channels, thereby preventing action potential propagation in nerve cells. They are well absorbed from mucosal membranes and commonly used for both surface and regional anaesthesia. Lidocaine solutions of 1% or 2% are generally used. Lidocaine is also available in combination with adrenalin/epinephrine, which counteracts the vasodilatory effect of local anaesthetics, and can therefore increase duration of action and reduce systemic absorption. It is important to choose carefully which preparation is needed, as adrenalin is harmful if given inappropriately (i.e. digital ring blocks). Great care should be taken to avoid accidental intravenous use, which can cause serious toxic effects (seizures, central respiratory and cardiac depression, bradyarrhythmias and hypotension). Initial symptoms of local anaesthetic toxicity are perioral tingling and parasthesia. If these occur, administration should be stopped. It is important to be aware of the maximum safe dose for the local anaesthetic being used. This is 3 mg/kg when lidocaine is used without adrenalin. A 1% solution contains 10 mg/mL, so for an average 70 kg patient the maximum dose would be approximately 20 mL of 1% lidocaine. Remember that this will be half the volume if 2% lidocaine is used. Larger volumes can be given if adrenalin is used. Local anaesthesia with lidocaine should occur within 2 minutes of skin infiltration, and lasts approximately 2 hours.

Other local anaesthetics such as bupivacaine are used for a range of local and regional anaesthesia, but this will normally be undertaken by specialists. Information is given in Table 37.1, but it is important to note that sources differ in estimating maximum doses; the most conservative doses are given in the table.

An approach to common prescribing requests I

Table 38.1 Guide to initial warfarin prescribing
(Source: NHS Grampian [based on the Fennerty regimen]. Reproduced with permission.)

Day	International normalised ratio (INR)	≤50 years	51-65 years	66-80 years	>80 years
1	<1.4	10	9	7.5	6
2	<1.6	10	9	7.5	6
	≥1.6	0.5	0.5	0.5	0.5
3	<1.8	10	9	7.5	6
	1.8–2.5	4–5	3.5–4.5	3–4	2.5–3
	2.6–3	2.5–3.5	2.5–3.5	2–2.5	1.5–2
	3.1–3.5	1–2	1–2	0.5–1.5	0.5–1.5
	3.6–4	0.5	0.5	0.5	0.5
	>4	0	0	0	0
4	<1.6	10–15	9–13	7.5–11	6–9
	1.6–1.9	6–8	5.5–7	4.5–6	3.5–5
	2–2.6	4.5–5.5	4–5	3.5–4.5	2.5–3.5
	2.7–3.5	3.5–4	3–3.5	2.5–3	2–2.5
	3.6–4	3	2.5	2	1.5
	4.1–4.5	Omit dose then give the following on day 5			
		1–2	0.5–1.5	0.5–1.5	0.5–1
	>4.5	Withhold warfarin until INR between 2–3 then restart on 0.5–1 mg			

The table gives advice for the first 4 days of warfarin initiation only, clinical judgement should be used from day 5 onwards.

When the INR result is towards the upper end of a range in the INR column, choose a dose towards the lower end of the range in dosage columns, and vice versa.

Decrease dose by one-third if patient has one or more of the following risk factors:
• Severe CCF
• Severe chronic obstructive pulmonary disease
• Concurrent treatment with amiodarone.

Prescribing at a Glance, First Edition. Sarah Ross. © 2014 John Wiley & Sons, Ltd. Published 2014 by John Wiley & Sons, Ltd.
Companion website: www.ataglanceseries.com/prescribing

General advice

Requests for treatment can come from many sources. In some instances, a particular treatment will be requested. It is essential that these requests are considered rather than merely obliged. You must familiarise yourself with the patient in order to prescribe safely and appropriately.

Can you prescribe warfarin for Mr Smith please?

General points

Warfarin is a difficult drug to use safely. Several facts are important to remember when prescribing it. Firstly, there is a huge inter-patient variability, with a maintenance dose range of around 0.5 mg to 15 mg. Secondly, warfarin has a long half-life. This means that dose changes can take 48 hours to be reflected in the international normalised ratio (INR). Thirdly, there are many drugs and foods which interact with warfarin, which should be taken into account when planning monitoring.

By convention, warfarin is usually taken at 6pm so that an INR can be checked first thing in the morning. Depending on the stability of the INR, monitoring can be as frequent as daily, but should be 8 weeks at the most.

Target ranges for different indications can be found in Chapter 28.

Initiating warfarin

The INR should be checked prior to starting warfarin to ensure that it is normal. Senior advice should be sought about the suitability of any patient without a normal clotting profile.

A loading regimen is needed because of the long half-life. This can be performed in several ways, depending on the urgency with which anticoagulation is needed, the location of the patient, and the patient's age. The most rapid method is to start with 10 mg of warfarin on the first day, then to give 10 mg, and then to use a dose as shown in Table 38.1. Variations on this method have been published and many hospitals have a protocol that can be followed. The danger with this method is over-anticoagulation, so initial dose adjustments are recommended in the elderly (5 or 6 mg instead of 10 mg). Check the INR each day and adjust these standard doses if needed. It is not uncommon to see a patient with an INR of >11 where the regimen has been used, but the INR has not been measured until day 3.

If slower anticoagulation is appropriate (e.g. for primary stroke prevention in atrial fibrillation, or initiation outside hospital) a regimen of 2 mg daily for a fortnight with an INR check at 7 days can be prescribed.

Maintenance dosing

In hospital, warfarin doses should be prescribed on a daily basis. This may mean that a prescriber may be asked to 'write up' warfarin for a patient that they do not know, based on the INR and last few doses on the drug chart. The first step is to know what the target INR is. If the INR is within target, it is reasonable to prescribe the patient's usual maintenance dose or the one that they have had over the last few days. If the INR is below target, an increase in dose may be needed. Be careful that the dose has not just been changed (in the last 48 hours) and there has not been enough time to see the INR increase. If this is not the case, a dose increase can be made. It is usually wise to do this in steps of 0.5 mg or 1 mg. Occasionally, if the INR is very low a larger dose increment may be appropriate.

If the INR is higher than target, either a dose reduction or temporarily withholding warfarin will be necessary. The British Haematological Society guidance for over-anticoagulation and bleeding can be found in Chapter 28. If there is no sign of bleeding and the INR is between 5 and 8, withholding warfarin for 1 to 2 days (or until INR <5) and reducing the maintenance dose by 1–2 mg should suffice. If the INR is below 5, a dose reduction should be sufficient. Remember to ensure that the INR is rechecked the following day.

Mrs Green is sore, can you prescribe some pain relief?

When asked to prescribe analgesia, it is wise to obtain additional information. What is the cause of the pain? How severe is the pain? What analgesia is the patient already receiving?

In addition, consider what can be done to deal with the cause of the pain. Be careful not to miss the pain of myocardial infarction in particular.

The WHO pain ladder (see Chapter 31) is a good place to start, whatever the situation. If the patient is not currently taking any analgesia, and the pain is mild to moderate, start with paracetamol. If the pain is moderate to severe, start further up the ladder.

If the patient is already taking analgesia, look at where they are on the pain ladder and go on to the next step.

Generally speaking, it is better to give regular analgesia, but on occasion a single dose, repeated when necessary, is reasonable. The route of administration should be oral if possible; however, parenteral routes can be used with some analgesics (i.e. paracetamol can be given intravenously, codeine intramuscularly, tramadol intramuscularly or intravenously, and morphine can be given subcutaneously, intramuscularly or intravenously).

Adjuvant analgesia with non-steroidal anti-inflammatory drugs is sensible if there is an inflammatory aspect (e.g. muscular or pleuritic pain) and if there is no contraindication.

Particular types of pain may respond to specific treatments (e.g. migraine can be treated with triptans, abdominal colic with hyoscine butylbromide).

Other adjuvants should normally be prescribed under senior or specialist advice.

An approach to common prescribing requests II

Table 39.1 Useful drugs at the end of life

Drug
Analgesics (e.g. paracetamol, strong opioid)
Anti-emetic, broad spectrum (e.g. levomepromazine)
Drug for agitation (e.g. midazolam)
Drug for respiratory secretions (e.g. hyoscine hydrobromide)

Can you prescribe anti-emetic for Mr Reid?

Again, additional information is needed. What is the cause of the nausea or vomiting? What treatment is the patient already receiving? Similarly, consider what can be done to deal with the underlying cause.

Consider whether additional pharmacological treatment is needed, or whether dealing with the cause will eliminate the symptoms. If additional treatment is needed, the probable cause of nausea/vomiting should be used to guide drug selection by matching an anti-emetic with an appropriate mechanism of action (see Chapter 30). A broad-spectrum anti-emetic may be helpful where the cause is unclear or more than one cause is present. At times, a combination of anti-emetics may be required. An anti-emetic 'ladder' is suggested, starting with one narrow spectrum agent and then moving to a second-line broad-spectrum or combination approach if required.

The vomiting patient should be given parenteral anti-emetic, whether intravenous, intramuscular or subcutaneous. The choice of route should be based on patient comfort as well as convenience. Remember that intramuscular injections are painful and may be avoidable. Patients who are suffering from nausea, but are not actively vomiting, may be able to take oral anti-emetics. In general, it is helpful to start off using regular doses, reducing these to as required when symptoms settle. As with all drugs, they should be stopped once the reason for nausea and vomiting has been dealt with.

Mrs Hobbs is agitated and I think she needs sedation

The management of confused and agitated patients in hospital settings is difficult. Pharmacological treatment may make the situation worse rather than better and can lead to adverse events. Where possible, try to reduce symptoms by dealing with the underlying cause (e.g. pain, urinary retention) and putting in place non-pharmacological measures.

Sedative drugs may be needed if the patient is a danger to themselves or to others. It is important that this is done in an ethical manner utilising the appropriate legal principles. Many hospitals will have a protocol that should be followed.

The main types of available medication are benzodiazepines and antipsychotics. Lorazepam and haloperidol are typical first-choice drugs.

Antipsychotics should not be used in patients with Lewy body dementia. They should also be avoided in cardiovascular disease if possible.

Where possible, offer drugs by the oral route. It may be necessary to use the intramuscular route. If more than one drug is to be used, do not mix in the same syringe as drugs may not be compatible. Use the lowest possible dose, and repeat if necessary after an interval, being careful not to exceed the maximum safe dose.

Flumazenil (the antidote to benzodiazepines) must be available to deal with respiratory depression caused by treatment. Remember this is more likely to happen with parenteral doses and in susceptible patients such as those with respiratory disease and the elderly.

Other important side effects that may occur include acute dystonia (where prescribing procyclidine may be necessary), haemodynamic disturbance (hypotension, bradycardia) and neuroleptic malignant syndrome (early signs are hyperthermia and/or rigidity).

Mr Stephen is dying. Do we need to prescribe anything?

A number of drugs can be useful in caring for the dying patient (Table 39.1). These can be prescribed as needed to manage the common symptoms of pain, agitation and difficult secretions. Obviously, there is a range of other drugs that may be needed and the patient may already be on strong analgesics. It is worth discontinuing any other drugs that are not providing symptom relief. The *British National Formulary* section on prescribing in palliative care is a good source of advice.

Not all patients experience pain during their last days; however, it is sensible to consider this eventuality. A small dose of morphine given subcutaneously can be helpful. Try to avoid the intravenous route as this will require the maintenance of intravenous access; also try to avoid the intramuscular route as this is painful. The oral route is usually not appropriate in the dying patient. Morphine is also a good treatment for breathlessness.

Terminal agitation is well recognised and distressing for patients and relatives. Small doses of subcutaneous midazolam can provide relief. Midazolam is also useful in preventing seizures.

The 'death rattle' caused by the build-up of oral secretions in the pharynx can be distressing. Hyoscine hydrobromide can be used to reduce this.

Medications may be given by continuous subcutaneous infusion using a syringe driver. Ensure that drugs are compatible if you are mixing medications. Diamorphine may be substituted for morphine if larger doses are needed as it is more soluble and can therefore be given in a much smaller volume. Some drugs should be avoided as they are an irritant when given subcutaneously (e.g. diazepam). Water for injection should normally be used to dilute drugs, although it can be an irritant at higher rates. Saline is more likely to cause drugs to precipitate within the syringe. Many hospitals will have a specialist palliative care team who will provide detailed advice about prescribing and support staff in this situation.

Prescribing at a Glance, First Edition. Sarah Ross. © 2014 John Wiley & Sons, Ltd. Published 2014 by John Wiley & Sons, Ltd.

Companion website: www.ataglanceseries.com/prescribing

Appendix
Cross references to *Prescribing Scenarios at a Glance*

Chapter in *Prescribing Scenarios at a Glance* (Ross)	Relevant case in *Prescribing Scenarios at a Glance* (Baker *et al.*)
Chapter 5 Reviewing current medicines	Chapter 18 A 58-year-old man who has low blood pressure
	Chapter 44 A 90-year-old woman on numerous medications
Chapter 14 Prescribing in liver disease	Chapter 33 A 47-year-old man who has developed an abnormal liver profile
	Chapter 49 A 49-year-old woman with chronic liver disease complaining of pain
Chapter 15 Prescribing in renal disease	Chapter 31 A 79-year-old woman with acute kidney injury
Chapter 16 Prescribing in children	Chapter 21 A 15-month-old girl with gastroenteritis
	Chapter 22 A 5-year-old boy with a painful right arm
	Chapter 23 A 12-hour-old boy with signs of sepsis
Chapter 17 Prescribing in the elderly	Chapter 44 A 90-year-old woman on numerous medications
Chapter 18 Prescribing in pregnancy and breast feeding	Chapter 40 A 23-year-old pregnant woman with pulmonary embolism
Chapter 19 How to write a drug prescription	Chapter 45 A 54-year-old woman with a peptic ulcer
Chapter 21 Therapeutic drug monitoring	Chapter 26 A 69-year-old woman being treated with gentamicin
	Chapter 41 A 31-year-old man with increased seizure frequency
Chapter 22 Dealing with adverse drug reactions	Chapter 24 A 60-year-old man who has developed a hot joint
Chapter 25 Using drugs for the gastrointestinal system	Chapter 37 A 69-year-old woman with constipation
Chapters 26, 27 and 28 Using drugs for the cardiovascular system I, II and III	Chapter 1 An 82-year-old woman who requires venous thromboembolism prophylaxis
	Chapter 4 An 84-year-old woman with atrial fibrillation
	Chapter 9 A 59-year-old man with acute pulmonary oedema
	Chapter 12 An 84-year-old man taking warfarin who has a headache
	Chapter 13 A 66-year-old man with acute coronary syndrome
	Chapter 48 A 70-year-old man with ST-elevation acute coronary syndrome
Chapter 29 Using drugs for the respiratory system	Chapter 10 A 24-year-old woman with acute asthma
	Chapter 14 A 67-year-old man with an exacerbation of COPD
Chapters 30 and 31 Using drugs for the neurological system I and II	Chapter 3 A 64-year-old man with severe acute abdominal pain
	Chapter 6 A 45-year-old woman with status epilepticus
	Chapter 16 A 60-year-old woman requesting night sedation
	Chapter 28 A 28-year-old woman with nausea
	Chapter 29 A 29-year-old man who is in pain following an operation
Chapter 32 Using drugs for infection	Chapter 5 A 32-year-old man with community-acquired pneumonia
	Chapter 7 A 27-year-old woman with suspected bacterial meningitis
	Chapter 32 An 85-year-old woman with hospital-acquired pneumonia
Chapters 33 and 34 Using drugs for the endocrine system I and II	Chapter 42 A 58-year-old man with diabetes mellitus treated with insulin
Chapter 35 Using drugs for the musculoskeletal system	Chapter 24 A 60-year-old man who has developed a hot joint
	Chapter 38 A 71-year-old man who has developed a tremor
	Chapter 39 An 81-year-old woman at risk of fragility fractures
Chapter 37 Using drugs in anaesthesia	Chapter 1 An 82-year-old woman who requires venous thromboembolism prophylaxis
	Chapter 30 A 49-year-old man due to undergo surgery
Chapters 38 and 39 An approach to common prescribing requests I and II	Chapter 3 A 64-year-old man with severe acute abdominal pain
	Chapter 16 A 60-year-old woman requesting night sedation
	Chapter 28 A 28-year-old woman with nausea
	Chapter 50 An 89-year-old man approaching the end of life

Prescribing at a Glance, First Edition. Sarah Ross. © 2014 John Wiley & Sons, Ltd. Published 2014 by John Wiley & Sons, Ltd.
Companion website: www.ataglanceseries.com/prescribing

Index

Note: Page entries in *italics* indicate figures; tables are noted with *t*; boxes are noted with b.

Prescribing at a Glance, First Edition. Sarah Ross. © 2014 John Wiley & Sons, Ltd. Published 2014 by John Wiley & Sons, Ltd.
Companion website: www.ataglanceseries.com/prescribing